100 Questions & Answers About Liver Cancer

FOURTH EDITION

Ghassan K. Abou-Alfa, MD, MBA
Memorial Sloan Kettering Cancer Center
New York, New York

Ronald P. DeMatteo, MD
Perelman School of Medicine at the University of Pennsylvania
Philadelphia, Pennsylvania

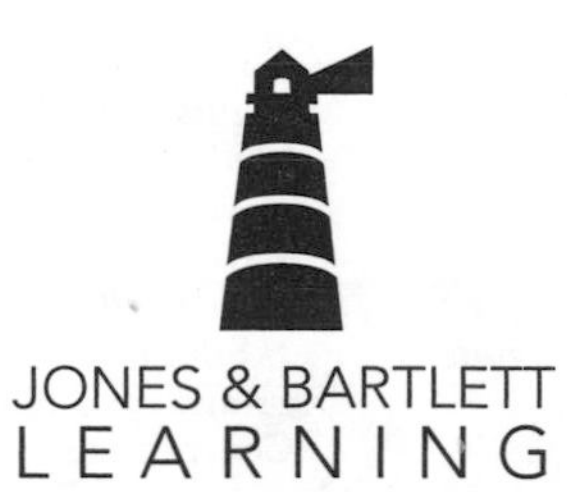

JONES & BARTLETT
LEARNING

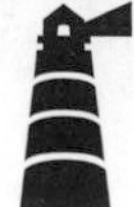

World Headquarters
Jones & Bartlett Learning
5 Wall Street
Burlington, MA 01803
978-443-5000
info@jblearning.com
www.jblearning.com

Jones & Bartlett Learning books and products are available through most bookstores and online booksellers. To contact Jones & Bartlett Learning directly, call 800-832-0034, fax 978-443-8000, or visit our website, www.jblearning.com.

Substantial discounts on bulk quantities of Jones & Bartlett Learning publications are available to corporations, professional associations, and other qualified organizations. For details and specific discount information, contact the special sales department at Jones & Bartlett Learning via the above contact information or send an email to specialsales@jblearning.com.

Production Credits
VP, Product Management: Amanda Martin
Product Manager: Teresa Reilly
Product Assistant: Christina Freitas
Product Assistant: Anna-Maria Forger
Production Manager: Daniel Stone
Marketing Manager: Lindsay White
Manufacturing and Inventory Control Supervisor: Amy Bacus
Composition: S4Carlisle Publishing Services
Cover Design: Scott Moden/Stephanie Torta
Rights & Media Specialist: John Rusk
Media Development Editor: Shannon Sheehan
Cover Image: Top Left: © imtmphoto/Shutterstock; (on alternative editions: Top Right: © Tetra Images/Getty; Bottom: Rocketclips, Inc./Shutterstock)
Printing and Binding: CJK Group, Inc.
Cover Printing: CJK Group, Inc.

ISBN13: 978-1-284-17219-5

6048

Printed in the United States of America
22 21 20 19 18 10 9 8 7 6 5 4 3 2 1

Contents

Preface *v*

Acknowledgements *vii*

Paul's Story *ix*

Part 1: The Basics *1*

Questions 1–4 provide information on all the basics about the liver and liver cancer, including:

- What is the liver?
- What is liver cancer?
- Are there different types of liver cancer?

Part 2: Risk Factors *5*

Questions 5–15 discuss the risks of developing liver failure (cirrhosis) and cancer, including:

- Is hepatocellular cancer common?
- Who is at risk for developing liver cancer?
- What is liver cirrhosis?

Part 3: Screening *17*

Questions 16–20 address who should be screened for liver cancer and what tests you might need, including:

- Who should be screened for liver cancer?
- Why is screening for liver cancer performed?
- What does screening entail?

Part 4: Diagnosis and Staging *21*

Questions 21–26 discuss what you would feel or complain of if you have liver cancer, as well as how your doctor will know if you have liver cancer, including:

- What are the symptoms of liver cancer?
- How is liver cancer diagnosed?
- What is cancer staging, and why is it relevant?

Part 5: Coping with the Diagnosis ***31***

Questions 27–32 answer questions about how to live with liver cancer, including:

- How long do people live with liver cancer?
- Does cirrhosis influence the treatment of liver cancer and the quality and length of life?
- What is supportive care?

Part 6: Treatment ***39***

Questions 33–78 offer information on all the therapies that are available to you to treat your liver cancer, including:

- Which treatment options are available for liver cancer?
- What is multidisciplinary care?
- What determines whether a tumor can be removed?

Part 7: Cancer-Related Practical Issues ***95***

Questions 79–85 address dealing with liver cancer on a day-to-day basis, including:

- I feel overwhelmed by all of the information that I am receiving. How do I make any decisions regarding my treatment?
- Will changing my diet alter my cancer?
- What is a mediport?

Part 8: Cirrhosis-Related Practical Issues ***105***

Questions 86–92 provide practical advice about managing all the complications of liver failure (cirrhosis), including:

- My legs and/or my abdomen are swollen. What can I do about it?
- What is meant when my platelets are low?
- I am vomiting or passing blood and coffee-ground material in my stool. What is causing this?

Part 9: Social and End-of-Life Issues ***113***

Questions 93–100 explore all the options that are available for support, or in case all therapies fail, including:

- Can my liver cancer be transmitted to my family?
- Can I work while getting treated?
- What if my doctors suggest stopping my current therapy?

Glossary ***123***

Index ***133***

Preface

Primary liver cancer is a very common form of cancer worldwide, often associated with existing liver failure or cirrhosis. Before being diagnosed with cancer, you may have been told a few years earlier that you had liver cirrhosis from hepatitis, alcohol use, morbid obesity and diabetes-associated fatty liver disease, or some other reason, and thus you may be at risk for developing primary liver cancer.

Dealing with liver cancer is a very complex matter, especially when it comes to medical care, as many specialists may be involved. You can expect to be treated by a gastroenterologist, a hepatologist regarding the liver cirrhosis, and many other specialists treating the cancer itself. These may include a surgeon, a medical oncologist, a transplant surgeon, an interventional radiologist, and a radiation therapist, among others.

One of the reasons we decided to write this book was to help you understand and coordinate your care among all those specialists. We also felt an important need for patients with liver cancer to understand all the available therapies, especially in view of the advent of new and emerging therapies. By the time we are writing this fourth edition, the number of treatments with positive outcome has multiplied by 6 and counting.

This book will also be of help in better understanding this cancer and all the signs and symptoms that may occur. We emphasize the management of symptoms like pain or leg swelling in an attempt to ensure comfort to all patients who are battling the disease. It is also an excellent resource for social issues that may arise as a result of the cancer. You will find information on how to handle fear, family concerns, work issues, and many other topics. Resources of all kinds, including websites, are listed.

We hope that you, your family, and friends find the answers and comfort you need through reading this book. Knowledge empowers, and as more advocates sound their voice, we believe this will help raise awareness in the battle against liver cancer.

Acknowledgements

The authors and publisher gratefully acknowledge the contribution provided by Mr. Paul Borkowski, whose comments appear in the front of the book.

The family of Paul J. Borkowski would like to extend their deepest appreciation to Dr. Abou-Alfa and the staff of Memorial Sloan Kettering Cancer Center (MSKCC). It was through their diligent and compassionate treatment that Paul enjoyed such excellent quality of life during the course of his journey with liver cancer. Paul was a valiant warrior who lived his life with faith and gratitude. His gigantic and empathetic heart touched many and he in turn indelibly touched the hearts of others. We who loved him salute him and wish him Godspeed!

Paul J. Borkowski passed away, peacefully, on June 28, 2008.

We would also like to extend our sincere appreciation to Mr. Sam Hou for graciously contributing his comments. Together with his family, Sam helped with the care of his father, Derson Hou, who was diagnosed with primary liver cancer in December 1999. While undergoing embolization and alcohol injection treatments at MSKCC, Derson experienced the daily joy of playing with his two new grandsons, Ryan and Samuel. Mr. Hou passed away, peacefully, in February 2004.

Ghassan K. Abou-Alfa, MD

Ronald P. DeMatteo, MD

Paul's Story

Around Thanksgiving of 2003, my annual battle with bronchitis and the usual upper respiratory complications began. I visited my primary care physician and started on my regular regimen of antibiotics. I had a history of emphysema and had contracted pneumonia on three separate occasions. In many ways, this felt familiar. Because I did not get any better in 2 weeks, we moved to the second step, an appointment with my pulmonologist. Something was different this time, because the usual tests did not produce the usual answers. I still had trouble catching my breath and was extremely fatigued all of the time, even though my cough was gone. My pulmonologist sent me to get a lung computed tomography (CT) scan. In the meantime, we made an appointment with my cardiologist to enlist his input about the problem. He must have seen something unusual in my symptoms because he recommended a whole-body CT scan with contrast. To be thorough, we made an appointment with my gastroenterologist.

The CT scan results were ready at the same time as my appointment with my gastroenterologist. He accessed the results while we were in his office. As it turned out, he was the one who told us the news. I can still remember sitting in his exam room when he came in with the results of my CT scan; I asked him to give us some good news. Instead, he said, "It seems that you have cancer." At that moment, the roof fell in on us. It was then that our journey with the "Big C" began.

Living on Long Island's South Shore, we proceeded to see an oncology group connected with South Side Hospital. The doctor was very nice and helpful. He had done his internship at Memorial Sloan Kettering Cancer Center and concurred with our plan to go to that institution for evaluation. He read the CT scan report that stated that I probably had a type of liver cancer known as hepatocellular carcinoma. His approach essentially consisted of offering palliative care. This approach seemed to be too passive; everyone we spoke with said since we live in Long Island, we had the option of going to the best, Memorial Sloan Kettering Cancer Center. This turned out to be very true in our case.

Our journey began in January 2004, with our first visit to Memorial Sloan Kettering Cancer Center. We had an appointment with a specialist to check the tumor near my lung. He assessed the tumors and said that it was basically a "slam dunk" to remove the tumor on my rib cage; however, he deferred to another specialist because the site of the liver tumor seemed to be primary. The liver surgeon told me that I was not a candidate for a transplant or surgery because my cancer had already metastasized. He added, "If you don't do anything, all you have is about a year to live." I did not appreciate hearing that because I had no intention of "doing nothing." We were then sent to Dr. Abou-Alfa at Memorial Sloan Kettering Cancer Center to explore the available options. From the first time we met Dr. Abou-Alfa, I liked him. He seemed to know his stuff! He was patient and kind, as well as very competent. His staff seemed very capable and dealt admirably with any and all questions that we had. It is very important to find the right doctor. Obviously, it is imperative to find someone who sees enough cases to develop skill and expertise. The type of cancer that I have is not too common in this country; consequently, the "neighborhood" doctors that I saw had an insufficient frame of reference for what my options actually were.

When you learn that you have cancer—no matter what type—your world seems to do a 180-degree turn. A lot of feelings seem to rise up—both good and bad! A lot of "wouldas, shouldas, and couldas" come up. As far as my life is concerned, the paths that some of these feelings and emotions took could have proven to be dangerous ground, leading to isolation, depression, or apathy. Luckily, I have the ability to surround myself with positive people and to keep my own outlook vital and upbeat. Many things in life just do not seem that important anymore or have to take a back seat to what is going on today.

At 57 years old, I found myself needing to take a long, hard look at my life. A number of really tough decisions would have to be made that would affect not only my life, but the lives of my family members as well. I had to reevaluate much in my life if I was to have any chance against this disease; I certainly was not going to lie down and give in to it.

First, I had to reevaluate my relationship with my God, whom I had taken for granted until this point. Also, my family and friends had to be seen in a different light. Since all of this came about, my family really has closed ranks around me, and I have learned who my real friends are. They are the ones who do not treat me as if I have the pox! I am not my cancer!

I also have come to believe in the power of prayer. Great feelings of peace and serenity can come from prayer and meditation. Every day, the prayer lines remain open. A number of angels—both seen and unseen—in my life have helped me with my burdens. Whether I am willing or able to ask for help, it seems that help is there anyway. I am truly grateful for this. All of my angels know who they are.

I also discovered many things that I still needed to do in my life in order to stand a chance with my disease. I had to retire from my job of 32 years with the U.S. Postal Service. That was a huge change in my daily routine, but it freed my time for treatment. Clouds often have silver linings, and retiring was an example of that truth for me. Education and knowledge became priorities for me, and they should for you, too. I discovered that there was much more to cancer than I as a layperson knew. I needed to learn as much as I could about my type of cancer. Questions such as these arose: Am I eligible for a liver transplant? If not, why? Why was I so constantly fatigued? What effect did my blood counts have on treatment? Decisions had to be made about whether to take part in a clinical trial or to go with standard treatment. I got a crash course in the phases of a clinical trial and how to negotiate websites to determine what trials were being offered. We spoke to researchers, doctors, and medical personnel around the country. After weighing all of the pros and cons, I decided to seek treatment at Memorial Sloan Kettering Cancer Center. The Internet was a great help as an overall resource, although it was overwhelming at times. Dr. Abou-Alfa and his very knowledgeable staff were there to answer any questions—and I had questions about everything! This book put together by Drs. Abou-Alfa and DeMatteo has been an invaluable tool in our search for answers to questions that we may have about my type of liver cancer (hepatocellular carcinoma). It does a great job of answering questions about why I got the type of liver cancer I have, how common it is, and where it comes from. This book covers other basics, such as how doctors test for hepatocellular carcinoma after the symptoms are detected. It discusses how to cope with the diagnosis and what treatment options are available. How important is it to discuss these options with your physician to determine which is best for you? This book takes an extremely concise and thorough look at all avenues that pertain to hepatocellular carcinoma, its causes and effects, and its diagnosis and treatment, as well as all of the practical issues right down to end-of-life issues.

To end on a good note: I am still here! It has been over a year, and I plan to keep on battling. I have found that I do not have to be alone in this battle, and neither does anyone else. My heartfelt thanks go to Dr. Abou-Alfa, Dr. DeMatteo, and their staff for all of their help and support. I am grateful to God for always being there. My deepest appreciation goes to my great wife and family and all of the angels in my life; their love and prayers are always accepted (humbly). To my fellow cancer patients, whose shared knowledge has made this journey possible and worthwhile: You have a special place in my heart. There is nothing like taking the journey with someone who knows what it feels like to walk in your shoes. I feel tremendous love and gratitude to each person in my circle of support. If I can help just one other person, I have done my part. Please do not ever give up hope, even when things seem to be at their darkest. A good attitude and a good sense of humor are golden tools to have in our corner. Try not to forget who is really in charge. I know I had a tendency to forget. I believe that is part of being human. Remember that prayer has the ability to move mountains and that miracles do happen!

Paul J. Borkowski

PART ONE

The Basics

What is the liver?

What is liver cancer?

Are there different types of liver cancer?

More . . .

Liver

An organ located in the upper right-hand side of the abdomen; responsible for making proteins and removing toxins and wastes from the body.

Proteins

Essential body substances that include enzymes, hormones, antibodies, and other substances that are critical for the functioning of the human body.

Bile

A collection of salts and proteins that is made by the liver and carried by the bile duct to the gallbladder and the intestine. Bile is green and gives feces their brown color.

Intestine

The part of the gastrointestinal tract between the stomach and rectum. The intestine helps digest food and regulate water, certain vitamins, and salts of the body.

1. What is the liver?

The **liver** is the largest organ in the body. It weighs approximately 1.5 kilograms (or slightly over 3 pounds). It resides in the upper abdomen on the right-hand side. Because most of the liver is underneath and protected by the right rib cage, you normally cannot feel it. The liver has numerous functions (**Box 1**). It is responsible for making many different **proteins**. It can be considered as the furnace of the body because it is the primary source of energy. It also acts as a filter to remove wastes and toxins from our blood. The liver makes **bile**, which empties into the **intestine**. Bile contains waste products as well as substances that help us to digest fat (Box 1).

2. What is liver cancer?

Like any other organ, the liver is made of basic elements called **cells**. A cell is the smallest structural unit of a living organism. Cells are born and die; thus, the body is always in need of new cells to replenish older and dead ones. This is a very tightly regulated phenomenon in the body. In certain instances, a cell becomes capable of

Box 1 Functions of the Liver

Stores energy in the form of sugar and carbohydrates.
Maintains normal blood sugar levels.
Breaks down fat.
Makes protein.
Stores vitamins A, D, and B_{12}.
Makes proteins that help blood clot.
Stores iron.
Removes drugs and toxins from the blood.
Produces cholesterol.
Makes bile.
Helps to protect your body from infection.

dividing in an uncontrolled fashion, and a **cancer** may then form and grow. Although the cells of a certain organ such as the liver are highly specialized and perform the tasks that are assigned to them, a **tumor** can lose some of its normal functions and/or acquire other new functions. One of the functions that cancer cells can acquire is the ability to grow and invade into the healthy parts of the same organ or a neighboring one. Cancer cells also can steal blood supply from normal tissue or form new blood vessels in order to grow larger. Cancer cells may even travel through the bloodstream to other organs or places in the body to establish new tumors. This process is called **metastasis**.

Cells
The smallest structural unit of a living organism that is capable of functioning independently.

Cancer
The uncontrolled replication of cells that leads to abnormal growth that may invade local organs or tissues or may travel to other places in the body.

Tumor
A cancerous growth.

Metastasis
The spread of cancer beyond its primary location.

3. Are there different types of liver cancer?

Two broad categories of liver cancer exist: primary and secondary (**Table 1**). **Primary liver cancer** means that the tumor originated in the liver. A tumor can start from any of the different types of cells that normally exist in the liver. **Hepatocellular cancer** is the most common type of primary liver cancer. It is also known as **hepatocellular carcinoma**, or **hepatoma** for short, and is often abbreviated HCC. Hepatocellular cancer (HCC) arises from **hepatocytes**, which are the cells that are responsible for most of the functions listed in Table 1.

Primary liver cancer
Cancer that originates within the liver.

Hepatocellular cancer
A type of primary liver cancer that originates in hepatocytes, a type of liver cell.

Hepatocellular carcinoma
A variant of hepatoma that occurs typically in young adults.

Table 1 Types of Liver Cancer

Primary liver cancer	Hepatocellular cancer Cholangiocarcinoma Mixed hepatocellular and cholangiocarcinoma Hepatoblastoma Gallbladder cancer
Secondary liver cancer	From colon, breast, pancreas, or other cancers

Hepatoma

Short name for hepatocellular cancer.

Hepatocytes

Liver cells.

Fibrolamellar hepatocellular carcinoma or fibrolamellar carcinoma

An independent and distinct form of liver cancer that occurs typically in young adults.

Cholangiocarcinoma

Cancer of the bile ducts inside (intrahepatic) or outside (extrahepatic) the liver.

Hepatoblastoma

A rare type of primary liver cancer that occurs in children.

Gallbladder

A storage tank for bile. It is attached to the liver. It squeezes the bile into your intestine when you eat a fatty meal.

Secondary liver cancer

Cancers that started in other organs of the body and have traveled to the liver.

There is a subtype of HCC called **fibrolamellar hepatocellular carcinoma** or, more precisely, **fibrolamellar carcinoma**. It makes up less than 1 percent of all HCCs. It tends to occur in young adults and is typically not associated with an underlying liver disease.

The other types of primary liver cancer are rare. **Cholangiocarcinoma** is a cancer that arises from the bile ducts within the liver (intrahepatic) or outside the liver (extrahepatic). Mixed hepatocellular and cholangiocarcinoma is a tumor that contains elements of both HCC and cholangiocarcinoma. **Hepatoblastoma** is a primary liver cancer that occurs in children. Cancer can also arise in the **gallbladder**. A variety of other very rare primary liver tumors exist.

Secondary liver cancer means that the cancer originated somewhere else in the body and then spread to the liver. Many cancers, like those of the colon, breast, and pancreas, can spread or metastasize to the liver. These patients do not have "liver cancer" in the way that doctors use the phrase. Instead, they have metastases to their liver. For example, if a breast cancer spreads to the liver, it is called metastatic breast cancer and is not referred to as liver cancer.

4. Which type of liver cancer is this book about?

In this book, we answer questions only about hepatocellular cancer, the most common type of primary liver cancer. This book is not written to answer questions about other types of primary or secondary liver cancers.

PART TWO

Risk Factors

Is hepatocellular cancer common?

Who is at risk for developing liver cancer?

What is liver cirrhosis?

More . . .

5. *Is hepatocellular cancer common?*

Almost 75 percent of all HCC cases occur in Asia. About 20,000 new cases of HCC are seen in the United States per year. The frequency of HCC in the U.S. and many other countries continues to increase, especially due to morbid obesity and diabetes-associated nonalcohol-associated fatty liver disease (also known as NAFLD; see Question 12). Worldwide, there are nearly a million new people affected per year. This is largely because of its association with **chronic viral hepatitis**, as explained in Question 8.

Chronic viral hepatitis

Continuous state of infection during which the liver continues to be inflamed and may ultimately cause cirrhosis and cancer.

Viral hepatitis

Inflammatory condition of the liver caused by an infection with a hepatitis virus.

6. *Who is at risk for developing liver cancer?*

Liver cancer rarely occurs spontaneously and for no apparent reason; in most instances, it starts because of an existing abnormality in the liver. Five main reasons exist for having an abnormal liver: (1) **viral hepatitis** B; (2) viral hepatitis C; (3) alcohol use; (4) obesity and **diabetes**; (5) other inherited **metabolic diseases** that affect the liver; and (6) environmental factors. These risk factors may exert their effect either through specific genetic changes, like in the instance of hepatitis B, or by causing severe damage to the liver that results in the development of liver failure also known as **cirrhosis**, or a combination of genetic changes and liver damage like in the instance of alcohol use.

Diabetes

A disease condition in which the body is unable to control sugar levels. In some instances, diabetes may lead to multiple complications and other diseases, and possibly primary liver cancer.

Metabolic diseases

Diseases in which the metabolism of a certain product may be impaired. They are usually genetically inherited.

7. *What is liver cirrhosis?*

Liver cirrhosis starts with fatty liver and is the replacement of many normal liver cells with scar tissue and a loss of the normal arrangement of the remaining liver cells. It generally takes years of liver damage for cirrhosis

Cirrhosis

Condition in which normal liver tissue is replaced with scar tissue. It is often associated with varied levels of loss of liver functions.

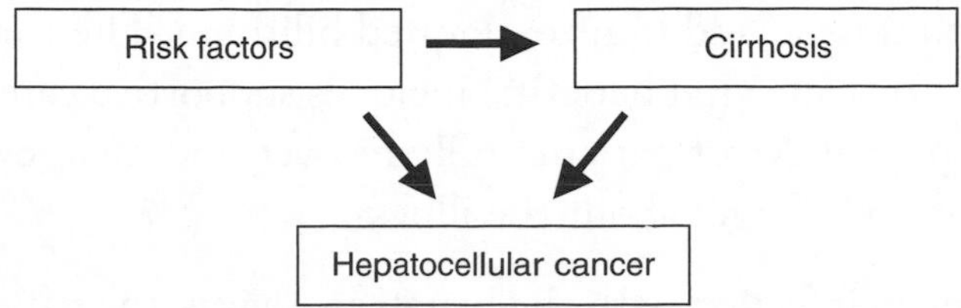

Figure 1 Relationship of risk factors for hepatocellular cancers to cirrhosis and cancer development.

to occur. Cirrhosis always affects the entire liver—not just one part of it. Cirrhosis is irreversible. Patients with severe cirrhosis and limited liver cancer may require and be eligible for a liver **transplantation** to get rid of cirrhosis. Patients with cirrhosis are at particular risk for developing HCC. Although cirrhosis is a common precursor to liver cancer, some patients develop HCC without ever having cirrhosis (see **Figure 1**).

Transplantation

The removal of a patient's entire liver and replacement with part or all of the liver from another person. The other person may be alive (live donor) or just deceased (cadaveric donor).

8. *What is viral hepatitis?*

The first risk factor for liver cancer that we consider is viral hepatitis. **Hepatitis** means inflammation of the liver. Some types of viruses that infect humans can damage the liver. The infection that may cause liver damage is called viral hepatitis. Viruses infect humans in order to divide and grow, because they cannot do so on their own. The most common hepatitis viruses were named A, B, and C, sequentially as they were discovered. Hepatitis A is caused by the hepatitis A virus, hepatitis B by the hepatitis B virus, and hepatitis C by the hepatitis C virus. **Acute viral hepatitis** means that a patient has become infected recently with the hepatitis A, B, or C virus. The patient may have a number of symptoms, including **fatigue**, loss of appetite, abdominal discomfort, and **jaundice** (yellow color of the eyes or skin due to elevated bilirubin). Usually, the patient will have abnormal liver

Hepatitis

Inflammation of the liver. It may be caused by a variety of agents, including viruses, excessive alcohol use, metabolic diseases, and environmental toxins.

Acute viral hepatitis

An active infection caused by a hepatitis virus.

Fatigue

Physical tiredness.

Jaundice

Yellow color of the eyes or skin due to elevated bile level (bilirubin) in the blood.

blood tests in addition to elevated bilirubin. The treatment of acute viral hepatitis includes supportive care of the patient. Most patients fully recover, and most even completely forget about the illness.

After an infection with the hepatitis A virus, the patient completely clears the virus from his or her body and is not at increased risk for cirrhosis or liver cancer. In contrast, some of the patients infected with the hepatitis B or C virus become chronically infected. In other words, they never completely remove the virus from their bodies. Patients with chronic hepatitis B or C are at risk for developing cirrhosis and all of its potential complications (see Question 22), including HCC.

9. What are the features of hepatitis B and chronic hepatitis B?

The chance of developing chronic hepatitis B depends on the age of the patient at the time of acute viral infection. Chronic disease will develop in approximately 90 percent of newborns, 25 percent of children, and 10 percent of adults. There are 1.2 million people with chronic hepatitis B in the United States and 350 million worldwide. The frequency of chronic hepatitis B is expected to decrease now that there is an effective vaccine against it. In some countries, hepatitis B is almost eradicated due to vaccination programs. However, many other countries still need a public health program to promote hepatitis B vaccination. In the United States, it is recommended that all children be vaccinated against hepatitis B. People may contract hepatitis B by coming in contact with blood or body fluids from an infected patient. For example, unprotected sexual contact with an infected individual may result in exposure to the virus. An infected mother may transmit hepatitis to her newborn child during birth. Perinatal exposure is most common in East Asia, whereas blood and sexual exposure are more common methods of transmission in Europe and North America. The highest incidence of hepatitis B, however, is in sub-Saharan Africa, where close encounter among children contributes to its high frequency in this area of the world. In Africa and Asia, hepatitis B infection is the predominant virus that contributes to the development of liver cancer. Especially if you are at risk, your doctor can perform blood tests to determine whether you have ever been exposed to hepatitis B in the past. If you have cleared the virus, then you are not contagious to others. Nevertheless, your family members should be tested because you were contagious during the acute viral infection and you may have transmitted the infection to others who were in close contact with you at that time. Blood tests can determine whether you have chronic hepatitis B. If you have chronic viral infection, then you are at risk for developing cirrhosis and/or liver cancer. Your family members should be tested. In addition, take precautions so that you do not transmit the virus to your family. Medications (e.g., **lamivudine** [Epivir], **entecavir** [Baraclude], **adefovirdipivoxil** [Hepsera]) can be taken to treat chronic hepatitis B. A liver specialist will determine whether you should be treated, and if so, with which drug. The goal of the treatment is to reduce the amount of virus in your body, and thus lower your risk of getting cirrhosis or cancer. Your chance of having liver cancer secondary to hepatitis B is about 0.5 percent per year. If you develop liver cancer secondary to hepatitis B, treatment of hepatitis B will still be an essential part of your care. A liver **biopsy** may be performed to determine whether you have signs of liver damage. You also will be advised to enter a screening program, as discussed later. In the instance of hepatitis B, liver

Lamivudine®, Barraclude®, Hepsera®

Antivirus drugs commonly used against hepatitis B.

Biopsy

The physical sampling of a piece of tissue. In patients with a suspected tumor, a biopsy is used to determine whether the patient has a cancer and what type of tumor it is. A biopsy is generally performed by passing a needle through the skin into a tumor.

cancer can develop shortly after the viral infection or years afterward.

My father was diagnosed with chronic hepatitis B about 3 to 4 years before his liver cancer was detected. His primary doctor had run a routine blood checkup and notified him that the hepatitis B screen came back positive. All of the immediate family members were then tested for the virus. My mother had developed protective antibodies, whereas my siblings and I tested negative for the virus. As a precaution, we then all received the newly developed vaccines for both hepatitis A and B.

Although we can never be 100 percent certain, my father most likely contracted the virus during a blood transfusion in his childhood in China and Taiwan before he immigrated to the United States. Even today, hepatitis and liver cancer are much more prevalent in Asian countries than in the West.

At the time of his hepatitis diagnosis, we were told there was nothing that could cure the hepatitis or reverse his liver cirrhosis. Later, we came across one possible treatment for hepatitis B: Epivir (lamivudine). In retrospect, I do not think that we realized that he was at a much higher risk for liver cancer as a result of the virus.

10. What are the features of hepatitis C and chronic hepatitis C?

Screening

Studies and evaluations that attempt to identify a predisease state or an early form of disease, aiming at controlling it before it becomes advanced.

Hepatitis C infection leads to chronic hepatitis in 55 to 85 percent of patients who are infected; 2.7 million patients have chronic hepatitis C in the United States. People who had a blood transfusion before 1992, prior to routine **screening** of blood products for hepatitis C, may have gotten hepatitis C. Today, it is extremely rare to get either form of chronic hepatitis from a blood transfusion. Contact with contaminated needles by intravenous drug users, healthcare workers, or people getting tattoos, is another mode of transmission. In the United States, hepatitis C viral infection is a major contributor to the risk of developing liver cancer.

Your doctor can perform blood tests to determine whether you have ever been exposed to hepatitis C in the past. If you have cleared the virus, then you are not contagious to others. Nevertheless, your family members should be tested because you were contagious during the acute viral infection. Unfortunately, there is still no vaccine against hepatitis C.

The blood tests also can determine whether you have chronic hepatitis C. If you have a chronic viral infection, then you have about a 20 percent risk for developing cirrhosis and a 5 percent risk for developing liver cancer. Your family members should be tested. Take precautions so that you do not transmit the virus to your family. A combination of ribavirin (Virazole, Rebetol) and interferon was originally used to treat chronic hepatitis C infection; nowadays hepatitis C can be cured with the use of new medications. The new drugs interfere with the proteins of the virus and prevent it from growing and spreading. There are several different options that your doctor may decide on based on what specific genetic type (or **genotype**) of hepatitis C you have and studying potential side effects that may be critical in your particular medical condition. Among those new drugs for hepatitis C are ledipasvir and sofosbuvir (Harvoni) for patients with genotype 1,4, 5, and 6; elbasvir and grazoprevir (Zepatier) for genotypes 1, 4, and 6; daclatasvir (Daklinza) with sofosbuvir (Sovaldi) for genotype 3; glecaprevir and pibrentasvir

Genotype
The genetic constitution of a specific virus or any organism.

(Mavyret), and ombitasvir, paritaprevir, ritonavir (Technivie) for genotype 4, among many others.

A liver specialist will determine whether you should be treated. The goal of the treatment is to cure you of the virus infection and thus eliminate your risk of getting cirrhosis or cancer. It is important to note that there are no data to justify treating you for the hepatitis C if you have already developed cancer. The safety and risks of such combination of anti-cancer therapy and treatment for hepatitis C still need to be established. A liver biopsy may be performed to determine whether you have signs of liver damage. You will be advised to enter a screening program, as discussed later. In many patients who develop liver cancer from chronic hepatitis, the cancer develops only after years of viral infection. For instance, cirrhosis and liver cancer can develop 10 to 30 years after exposure to hepatitis C.

Hepatitis C infection leads to chronic hepatitis in 55 to 85 percent of patients who are infected.

11. How does alcohol use affect my liver?

Alcoholic liver disease

Liver cirrhosis caused by excessive alcohol ingestion.

Fatty liver

Condition in which fat accumulates in the liver because of a liver illness caused by one of several diseases (e.g., viral hepatitis).

Alcohol use is another risk factor for liver cancer. **Alcoholic liver disease** is caused by chronic and excessive ingestion of alcohol. The quantity and duration of alcohol intake are the most important factors. An average of 60 to 80 grams of alcohol intake per day puts a person at high risk for developing liver disease. This amount is equivalent to an average of six cans of beer, 23 ounces of wine, or 6 ounces of 80 percent proof spirits. A smaller amount of alcohol ingestion in women can lead to cirrhosis and thus liver cancer. Another consequence of alcohol on the liver is the development of a **fatty liver**, which can occur in over 90 percent of heavy drinkers and binge drinkers.

12. What is the association between obesity, diabetes, and liver cancer?

Researchers have discovered that diabetic patients have a slightly increased probability of developing liver cancer compared to those who do not have diabetes. Other researchers also found that patients who are severely obese have an increased chance of developing and dying from liver cancer. Diabetes and severe obesity are closely associated with a type of liver abnormality called **nonalcoholic fatty liver disease** (also known as NAFLD), which might lead to **nonalcoholic steatohepatitis** (also known as NASH), cirrhosis and ultimately liver cancer. This is an emerging concept that has not yet been proven. If you are obese or have diabetes, your doctor will discuss these potential risk factors and any precautions that should be taken. Unfortunately, obesity and diabetes continue to be on the rise in the United States.

Nonalcoholic fatty liver disease

Disease that leads to the development of fatty liver by injuries other than excessive alcohol use.

13. What are the inherited metabolic diseases that affect the liver?

Several rare inherited diseases can cause liver damage and may lead to cirrhosis and/or liver cancer. One of these diseases is called **hemachromatosis**. It leads to the accumulation of a mineral in the liver and results in cirrhosis, which increases the risk of liver cancer. Hemochromatosis is an illness of increased iron absorption and deposition in many organs of the body, including the liver. The disease is inherited and is most commonly seen among northern Europeans or their descendants. People who are affected can live a normal life, but many (especially men) start to have symptoms around age 40 years. Affected individuals may start to feel tired and weak and may acquire a shiny tan to their skin in the absence of

Nonalcoholic steatohepatitis

Progression from nonalcoholic fatty liver disease to cirrhosis and potentially cancer.

Hemochromatosis

A hereditary disease that leads to excessive accumulation of iron in the body and may cause liver disease and ultimately primary liver cancer.

sun exposure because of iron deposition in the skin. People of northern European ethnicity may know of family or relatives who have blood drawn very frequently. This is done to reduce the amount of iron in the body because blood contains a lot of iron. If you have the symptoms just listed or have family members affected by this disease, you might need to be screened for hemochromatosis. The increased deposition of iron in the liver may lead to liver cirrhosis, liver failure, and cancer.

There are multiple other genetic diseases that might cause inflammation in the liver (hepatitis) and cirrhosis and therefore can lead to the development of liver cancer. Some of these diseases are listed in **Box 2**.

Wilson's disease

An inherited disease of impaired copper metabolism.

Box 2 Genetic Diseases that May Cause Liver Cancer

Hemochromatosis
Wilson's disease
Alpha-1 antitrypsin deficiency
Primary biliary cirrhosis
Porphyria cutanea tarda
Types 1 and 3 glycogen storage disease
Galactosemia
Citrullinemia
Hereditary tyrosinemia
Familial cholestatic cirrhosis
Familial polyposis coli
Ataxia telangiectasia
Biliary atresia
Congenital hepatic fibrosis
Neurofibromatosis
Situs inversus
Fetal alcohol syndrome
Budd-Chiari syndrome

14. Which environmental factors may cause liver cancer?

Exposure to **aflatoxins** is associated with liver cancer. Aflatoxins are produced by two **fungi**: *Aspergillus flavus* and *Aspergillus parasiticus*. These fungi usually grow on grains. This is especially hazardous in certain African regions and in southern China. These fungi are responsible for most food spoilage in these tropical regions. Liver toxicity from aflatoxins may lead to the development of liver cancer. Obviously, there is a certain level of aflatoxins needed to cause such injury to the liver. Minute amounts of aflatoxins are present in many crops, but their level is far below one that is considered dangerous.

Aflatoxins

A group of molds that contaminate stored food supplies and may lead to cirrhosis and ultimately liver cancer.

Fungus

A type of organism that can cause an infection.

Certain chemicals, such as nitrites, hydrocarbons, solvents, and organochlorine pesticides may also cause liver cancer. Your doctor and possibly an environmental health specialist may need to evaluate you carefully if you have been exposed to these chemicals. Other factors still may need to be considered because a definitive relationship has not been proven for each type of chemical exposure.

15. How can I reduce my risk of getting liver cancer?

If you already have chronic hepatitis, then you should consult with your doctor about taking medication to help clear the virus from your body. You also should avoid behavior that may expose you to another type of hepatitis virus. For instance, if you have chronic hepatitis B and you become infected with hepatitis C, your risk of liver cirrhosis and liver cancer is substantially increased; thus you have to seek treatment and potentially cure of the hepatitis C. Obviously, if you use

A number of things can be done to lower the risk of getting liver cancer.

excessive alcohol, seek medical help to treat your dependency. Also, excessive alcohol use should be avoided if you have chronic hepatitis. If you have an inherited disease that puts you at higher risk of liver cancer, work closely with your doctor to optimize the treatment of your condition. Patients who have diabetes or severe obesity should be under close medical attention and abide by their prescribed medical and fitness regimens. Similarly, if you have concerns regarding environmental exposures, you should consult with an environmental medicine physician and possibly a liver specialist. If you develop liver cancer, it would be very important to be treated for certain conditions (e.g., hepatitis B or excessive alcohol use), because reducing those risks may improve your liver function and help you avoid developing another primary liver cancer.

PART THREE

Screening

Who should be screened for liver cancer?

Why is screening for liver cancer performed?

What does screening entail?

More . . .

16. Who should be screened for liver cancer?

From a practical standpoint, a person who carries any of the previously discussed risk factors should be screened for liver cancer. For example, individuals with chronic hepatitis B or C infection should be regularly evaluated by a physician for the development of liver cirrhosis and liver cancer. This also applies to individuals with a history of excess alcohol ingestion, especially if they have liver problems; patients with a family history for any genetic disease that carries a risk of developing liver cancer; and patients with an environmental risk, especially if they already have evident liver problems. Although there are no clear recommendations for screening, if you are diabetic and obese, many physicians believe that you should be followed very closely. This is especially true if you already have a fatty liver as your doctor can determine by blood tests and possibly a liver biopsy (if indicated). It is particularly important to mention again that no specific guidelines exist regarding screening, so you should discuss your situation with your physician to assess the benefits and risks of any recommended screening tests.

17. Why is screening for liver cancer performed?

The reason to screen patients who are considered to be at high risk of developing a liver cancer is that if a liver cancer does occur, the tumor more likely will be detected when it is small and before it has spread to other parts of the liver or elsewhere in the body. In other words, screening may allow detection of a cancer in an early stage. Otherwise, many patients with liver cancer may have advanced disease by the time they have symptoms and seek medical attention. This happens for two reasons. First, the liver does not sense pain very well. Only the outside lining of the liver (called the **liver capsule**) has **nerve** fibers. Therefore, a tumor inside the liver may not cause any symptoms of pain. Second, the liver has a tremendous functional reserve. As a result, even an advanced tumor may not alter the normal function of the liver and may not cause any abnormalities on routine blood work. In general, most doctors recommend screening because they believe that patients with early-stage liver tumors have the best chance of being cured with treatments such as surgery. Nevertheless, the precise benefit of finding cancers when they are small has not been definitively proven.

Liver capsule

The outside lining of the liver. It is the only part of the liver that can trigger a sensation of pain.

Nerve

A type of tissue in the body that can transmit sensations such as pain, pressure, or temperature.

18. What does screening entail?

This is a controversial issue. However, most physicians recommend an **ultrasound** of the liver and a blood test to measure an **alpha-fetoprotein**, known as AFP. An ultrasound uses sound waves to image internal organs. This is the same test that is used to look at fetuses in pregnant women. During an ultrasound of the liver, a technician or doctor places a probe over your liver, which is located in the upper right portion of your abdomen. Typically, the test is easy and painless and does not involve any injections or **radiation** exposure. You may feel some pressure at the site being evaluated as the probe is pushed close to your body. Some doctors may prefer to use a different type of radiologic test such as a **computed tomography (CT) scan** or **magnetic resonance imaging (MRI)**, both of which are described in Question 23.

Ultrasound

The use of ultrasonic waves to view images of an internal body structure.

Alpha-fetoprotein

A blood marker that may be elevated in primary liver cancer.

Radiation

A ray of powerful energy that is emitted from a radioactive material.

Computed tomography (CT) scan

A form of x-ray images in which acquired images are constructed by computer to form cross-sectional images of the body.

AFP (alpha-fetoprotein) is a protein that appears in the blood of approximately 60 percent of patients with liver cancer. Therefore, a positive blood test for AFP can be an

Magnetic resonance imaging (MRI)

A form of radiologic imaging that uses magnetic fields to produce electronic images of the inner parts of the human body.

early indicator that a patient has a liver cancer. However, AFP alone is insufficient as a screening tool, because certain liver cancers do not secrete or produce AFP. Thus, a normal AFP level could be misleading, and not all doctors agree to screen for AFP. Also, not every elevated AFP level indicates the presence of liver cancer. Many other situations exist where AFP can be elevated. For example, it is normally elevated in pregnancy. AFP also can be elevated in other cancers such as testicular cancer and stomach cancer. Screening for liver cancer relies on a comprehensive assessment and evaluation conducted by your physician and does not rely on any single test.

19. How often should a patient who is at high risk of liver cancer be screened?

This unsettled issue currently is being studied; thus, there is no universal consensus of opinion at this time. Many physicians recommend that a liver specialist evaluate patients who are at high risk of developing liver cancer every 3 to 6 months. The doctors generally recommend liver blood tests and an AFP level twice a year and a liver ultrasound once a year.

20. What should be done if a screening test suggests that a patient has a liver cancer?

If an ultrasound shows or suggests a liver mass and/or if the AFP is elevated, further tests will be required. A CT scan or an MRI is often used to evaluate abnormal ultrasound findings or an elevated AFP. If an abnormality is confirmed, you should be evaluated by a multidisciplinary group of doctors and other healthcare professionals, as discussed in Questions 29 and 34.

PART FOUR

Diagnosis and Staging

What are the symptoms of liver cancer?

How is liver cancer diagnosed?

What is cancer staging, and why is it relevant?

More . . .

21. What are the symptoms of liver cancer?

As discussed in Question 17, by the time a liver cancer causes symptoms, many patients already have advanced disease. The most common symptom is a dull abdominal ache below the right rib cage, where the liver is located. The pain sometimes may travel to the right shoulder. Patients might lose weight, lose their appetite, or have a fever that is not explained by any infection. On physical examination, your doctor might detect that your liver is enlarged or even feel a mass in the liver. Some patients have no symptoms, and a tumor is detected incidentally on screening tests or during blood work or radiologic tests performed to evaluate other conditions.

22. Are the symptoms of liver cancer different in a patient with cirrhosis?

In many instances, cirrhosis is the breeding ground for the development of liver cancer. Often, liver cancer can present as worsening cirrhosis. The liver as a large organ can compensate for cirrhosis, the causes of which were discussed previously. However, sometimes the cirrhosis worsens, and the liver fails. One reason for this liver failure is that as the liver tumor replaces the noncancerous liver, which is already abnormal from cirrhosis, the patient no longer has adequate liver function reserves. Thus, a liver tumor may cause worsening cirrhosis.

Abdominal distention

Bulging of the belly.

Ascites

An abnormal accumulation of fluid in the abdomen.

Peripheral edema

Excessive accumulation of fluids in the legs that leads to swelling.

Several things normally occur in cirrhosis, any of which can be worsened by a liver tumor (**Box 3**). A patient may have **abdominal distention** with fluid buildup in the abdomen called **ascites**. Fluid buildup can also occur in the legs and is called **peripheral edema**. Patients may

Box 3 Complications of Cirrhosis

Ascites
Peripheral edema
Jaundice
Mental confusion
Portal hypertension
Variceal bleeding

acquire a yellowish discoloration to their skin and eyes, called jaundice. Jaundice also results in a lighter color of stools because bile is not released as well into the intestine to give stool its normal dark color. The pigments spill over to the blood and are partially filtered by the **kidneys**, resulting in dark or tea-colored urine. Further decompensation of the liver might lead to its inability to metabolize or get rid of different toxins. These might accumulate in the body, including the brain, and might cause mental confusion, drowsiness, forgetfulness, or sleepiness called **encephalopathy**. This decompensation associated with liver cancer growth also can be explained by the possible direct growth of the cancer into the blood supply of the liver. Clogged vessels by the tumor or a severely cirrhotic liver might build up pressure on the vessels on the outside of the liver. This is called **portal hypertension**. This buildup of pressure could lead to abnormally swollen or dilated small vessels that ultimately may break and bleed. A typical place for this bleeding to occur is in the stomach or esophagus. A patient might experience bloody or dark vomiting or might notice black stools. Sometimes the patients may not notice the bleeding but will become tired. These **variceal bleeds** warrant immediate medical evaluation.

Kidneys

Two organs located in the abdomen that are responsible for water and electrolytes balance, and that help excrete body metabolites through urine.

Encephalopathy

An altered sense of consciousness. It may occur when the liver is not working well. The patient may seemed confused or have inappropriate social behavior. It may vary in severity from day to day.

Portal hypertension

Increased pressure within the veins of the liver, which can lead to poor liver function, increased size of the spleen, and consequently, a low platelet count, or varices (dilated veins of the stomach or esophagus).

Variceal bleed

An actively bleeding varix, which is a dilated vein.

23. How is liver cancer diagnosed?

If a patient is suspected of having a liver tumor based on screening tests or experiencing new symptoms, he or she will require a more definitive imaging test, such as a CT scan or an MRI. A CT scan is a computer-generated picture of multiple x-rays of the body taken at different angles—the collection of which make up "sliced" pictures of the human body. An MRI makes a similar picture but uses a magnetic field instead of radiation. Although MRIs sound more appealing because they do not require radiation, the radiation exposure from CT scans is considered safe, especially at the frequency that CT scans are required to follow your cancer. Both techniques require an injection of a material given through the vein called contrast that helps differentiate the different structures of the body. For example, a CT scan contrast can highlight blood vessels and primary liver tumors, especially since the latter have a number of blood vessels that supply them. If you were to get a CT scan, it is recommended that you have a triphasic or four-phase CT scan, which can help evaluate primary liver tumors at different times of the flow of blood through the liver and thus help better define the tumor. A CT scan may be contraindicated if you previously developed a severe allergic reaction to the contrast material. Usually, pretreatment with steroids and diphenhydramine (Benadryl) can help prevent allergic reactions if you have had previous mild reactions to contrast agents. With a CT scan, you also may be required to drink a contrast solution to help highlight the stomach, intestines, and bowels. A patient who is claustrophobic may have difficulty with an MRI because he or she will have to lie still in a confined tube during the test. Patients who have certain metal parts in their body, such as an artificial knee, may not be eligible for an MRI. Usually a patient is given a questionnaire to determine whether he or she can obtain an MRI. Your doctor will advise which test you should undergo, as each one provides slightly different information.

A mass or multiple masses in the liver may be noted. It is important to mention that liver cancer can invade local blood vessels and block them. It also can invade local **lymph nodes** or even spread to other organs. A good imaging study should usually identify these possibilities. Three general growth patterns of HCC exist inside the liver. The tumor can grow as a well-circumscribed nodule. The tumor can be more invasive and grow diffusely without any apparent boundaries in an area of the liver. HCC also can grow as multiple nodules scattered within the liver.

Lymph nodes
Small bodies along the lymphatic system that supply a special kind of fighter white blood cells called lymphocytes to the bloodstream. They are also responsible for removing bacteria and foreign particles from the lymph. Lymph nodes may be invaded by cancer and may also help transmit cancer to other sites of the body. Lymph nodes are also known as lymph glands.

An AFP blood test will be obtained if it has not been performed already. Although an elevated AFP (normal is usually 0 to 15 ng/ml) may suggest the presence of liver cancer, it is nonspecific and may reflect another medical condition in the body as discussed previously. More importantly, some liver cancers do not cause an elevated AFP. Thus, an AFP blood test by itself is not diagnostic but is complementary to the radiologic and blood tests that your doctor might request. An elevation of AFP above 400 ng/dl along with two different imaging tests (for example, a CT scan and an MRI) that show a tumor is considered virtually diagnostic of a liver cancer in the appropriate clinical setting. This, however, is not necessarily true and can incorrectly diagnose certain medical conditions as liver cancer in about 15 to 20 percent of the cases (see Question 24). The degree of AFP elevation does not necessarily reflect the amount of disease present because even small tumors can produce substantial amounts of the protein.

If a patient is suspected of having a liver tumor based on screening tests or experiencing new symptoms, he or she will require a more definitive imaging test, such as a CT scan or an MRI.

Prognostic

A blood test, sign, or other element that helps predict the likely course of the cancer.

Radiologists

Doctors who specialize in interpreting x-rays, CT scans, MRIs, and other radiologic tests.

An AFP blood test by itself is not diagnostic but is complementary to the radiologic and blood tests that your doctor might request.

The magnitude of the AFP level can depend on the cause of the tumor. It is known that hepatitis B may lead to high AFP levels independent of the extent of the cancer, while hepatitis C–related liver cancer may be quite extensive and yet have limited or no AFP expression at all. There is a debate in regard to the **prognostic** value of AFP as well. Despite how advanced the technology seems, CT and MRI scans are not always precise. Depending on the exact machine and the skill of the operator, the scans can sometimes be fuzzy and open to interpretation. Also, sometimes small spots or lesions can show up on the scan that may or may not be cancerous. Ask the **radiologist** for copies of the report and then ask your doctor for his or her opinion. Sometimes, serial scans are needed to decipher whether an abnormality on a scan is actually a tumor.

24. Is a biopsy required for diagnosis?

As with most other cancers, the ultimate proof that you have a cancer depends on a biopsy, which is performed by sampling a piece of the tumor. In some instances, a surgeon might elect to remove a tumor without obtaining a biopsy of the tumor. This decision would be built on a collection of evidence to proceed directly to surgery without first obtaining a biopsy. For instance, if you have an AFP of greater than 400 ng/dl and a mass that is consistent with an HCC on a CT or an MRI, then a presurgical or pretransplant biopsy may not be necessary. Generally, if you are treated with a local therapy (e.g., embolization) (see Question 33), a biopsy is done prior to the procedure. A biopsy also is performed before starting **chemotherapy** or **biologic therapy** to treat a cancer. This confirmation is important because sometimes other conditions can masquerade as HCC. There may be serious side effects that

Chemotherapy

Chemical agents that are used to treat cancer.

Biologic therapy

Novel agents aimed at specific targets used to treat cancer.

occur with systemic therapy, so it is important to make sure the diagnosis is correct. Furthermore, HCCs are not all the same and they differ genetically between different patients. In the future, having certain tests that may be done on a sample of your tumor may help define certain therapies that may be more beneficial for your specific primary liver cancer.

A liver biopsy typically is obtained via a needle that is placed through the skin. To ensure the safety and adequacy of the sample, a needle biopsy usually is performed under radiologic guidance using either an ultrasound or a CT scan. The procedure itself is relatively safe and causes only minor discomfort. A **local anesthetic** will be injected into your skin to minimize any pain. The doctor performing the procedure will discuss the potential complications of a biopsy. These are rare but include the possibility of bleeding or infection. In most instances, you can leave on the same day. Contrary to some misconceptions, liver biopsies do not cause worsening of the cancer. However, in certain instances of advanced cirrhosis and a high risk of bleeding, a liver biopsy may be contraindicated. Your doctor should discuss the benefits and risks of obtaining a biopsy.

Local anesthetic

Numbing medication that is injected directly at the site where a procedure is to be performed.

Pathology laboratory

The section of the hospital in which a pathologist works and where tissue specimens are analyzed.

25. What can you learn from a biopsy?

The tissue obtained by a biopsy typically is sent to a **pathology laboratory**, where it is sliced into very thin cuts that are applied to 3 × 1–inch glass slides, known as **pathology slides**. The very thin cuts are stained with different chemicals that color various structures. A **pathologist** then looks at these under a microscope. A pathologist can view the cancerous cells and estimate how aggressive they are. Because many cancers can metastasize the liver, the pathologist also needs to confirm

Pathology slides

3 × 1–inch glass slides on which tissue from a biopsy or a surgical specimen is placed.

Pathologist

A doctor who specializes in the diagnosis of diseases of the body by evaluating biopsies from the disease site, like cancer.

that the tumor is indeed HCC and not another primary liver cancer or a secondary liver cancer. The pathologist also can tell if there is cirrhosis and how advanced it is. A typed **pathology report** is generated based on the findings of the pathologist.

Pathology report

A typed report issued by a pathologist that describes the results of the analysis of a biopsy or surgical specimen.

Genetic testing may also take place. Physicians nowadays may order or recommend a next-generation sequencing (NGS) test, which allows for a thorough look at a certain number of **genes** that can help with diagnosis, inheritance, and therapy choices. The genetic testing at Memorial Sloan Kettering is an FDA-authorized test that provides information on close to 450 genes.

Genes

A unit of heredity that is transferred from a parent to offspring and is held to determine some characteristic of the offspring.

26. What is cancer staging, and why is it relevant?

Patients and physicians alike need a way to communicate the status of the cancer. Liver cancer differs from other cancers by having two components: the cancer itself and the commonly associated liver cirrhosis (see Question 7).

The cancer itself can involve one or more sites in the liver, blood vessels in and around the liver, lymph nodes close to the liver, and distant organs such as the bone. To be able to communicate this information and decide on a plan of care, physicians use a **staging system**. In liver cancer, the first step in staging a tumor is to determine whether it consists of one or more tumors, its size or sizes, whether it involves any blood vessels, and whether it has any further local extension. This is given a T (for tumor) score. Lymph nodes are evaluated next and are given an N (for node) score, and finally, any disease that has spread to other sites is given an M (for metastasis) score. Combining the T, N, and M scores assigns a stage to the cancer that ranges between I and IV. Stages I and II indicate a tumor that is confined to the liver.

Staging system

A set of definitions that allows physicians to define the extent of a certain cancer and recommend therapy accordingly.

Stage III is subdivided into groups A, B, or C and includes cancers that invade major blood vessels, other organs in close proximity to the liver, or lymph nodes. Stage IV disease is any disease that has spread beyond the liver or the region of the liver.

In addition to the staging of the cancer, an evaluation or a score of the extent of cirrhosis is important. This can be done through different scoring systems. The Child-Pugh scoring system is widely used and can categorize the extent of cirrhosis you might have. The Child-Pugh scoring system is generated by assessing a combination of physical examination and laboratory variables. It classifies patients with cirrhosis into three categories: A, B, and C. Child-Pugh A patients have the least cirrhosis, and C have the most cirrhosis. More complex scoring systems that can assess both the extent of the cancer and cirrhosis are used nowadays. There is, however, no consensus as to which is the most valuable. Hepatologists commonly use the BCLC system. Surgeons and transplant surgeons use the MELD (see Question 47) and Okuda scoring systems. **Oncologists** use the CLIP, CUPI, and ALBI. The CLIP is more commonly used in Europe and North America, while the CUPI is more commonly used in southeast Asia.

Oncologists

Medical doctor specialists who treat cancer.

It is important to note that though cancer staging and the extent of cirrhosis give a fairly accurate assessment on outcome and prognosis, some other variables that are not as well defined may also play a role. For example, two patients with stage IV cancer may not necessarily have the same outcome, probably because of different biologic variables that may render one more or less aggressive than the other. While the pathology examination may help assess some of those aspects, other factors may not be apparent until you start treatment and it becomes clear how you are responding.

PART FIVE

Coping with the Diagnosis

How long do people live with liver cancer?

Does cirrhosis influence the treatment of liver cancer and the quality and length of life?

What is supportive care?

More . . .

27. How long do people live with liver cancer?

This is a difficult question, and no simple answer is available. How someone will do depends on the stage of his or her cancer, his or her general medical condition, the health of the part of his or her liver not affected by cancer, and the treatment options for which he or she is eligible. Your doctor can give you an idea of how you may do. In other words, your doctor can estimate your survival based on how large groups of patients have done in the past. However, even experienced physicians often cannot accurately determine how one particular patient may fare. Building a close relationship with your physicians is important to help deal with your fears that might grow after being diagnosed with cancer. Your doctors should be in a position to recommend the best approach of therapy based on the stage of the disease. This, by itself, might influence the possibility of cure and survival.

28. Does cirrhosis influence the treatment of liver cancer and the quality and length of life?

In contrast to many other cancers, liver cancer is often two diseases in one. Cirrhosis by itself contributes to the development of cancer and directly affects the level of function of the liver. A cirrhotic liver will be unable to synthesize or make the essential proteins and bile. It also will fail to metabolize or break down the different compounds that go through the liver. A badly cirrhotic liver might affect survival and can actually be a worse problem than the cancer it harbors. Even therapeutic decisions regarding the cancer might be influenced by the degree of cirrhosis. Although a cancer specialist may treat a patient primarily for liver cancer, often a liver specialist (**hepatologist**) may need to be involved. Cirrhosis is graded using different criteria. One of the more commonly used grading systems is the **Child-Pugh score**, as discussed previously. This score assesses the synthetic and metabolic functions of the liver.

Hepatologist
A liver disease specialist.

Child-Pugh score
A score used to assess the level of cirrhosis.

29. What is supportive care?

The diagnosis of liver cancer may have a severe impact on a patient. In addition to the cancer and the cirrhosis (if present), other concerns including nutrition and pain control might be present. This is not to understate the psychologic, social, and financial impact. A person who is working and is found to have liver cancer might have his or her lifestyle come to a halt. As much as this might seem very discouraging, most doctors believe that a multifaceted supportive team approach might alleviate many, if not all, of the common concerns. In addition to the multidisciplinary care approach (see Question 34), you also may need the help of pain specialists, nutritionists, psychiatrists, and social workers. A typical comprehensive cancer center has a team of several types of doctors and healthcare workers. In addition, patient support groups and **integrative medicine** may be helpful. Integrative medicine is a growing discipline that addresses the emotional, social, and spiritual needs of patients and their families. This helps to increase self-awareness and enhances well-being.

How someone will do depends on the stage of his or her cancer, his or her general medical condition, the health of the part of his or her liver not affected by cancer, and the treatment options for which he or she is eligible.

30. Should a patient get a second opinion?

Patients who are diagnosed with cancer often obtain a second opinion. Most doctors encourage that, because the second opinion may provide the patient with

Integrative medicine
A discipline that is used to treat patients using modern science and alternative medicine.

additional information. You may actually receive conflicting opinions about what you should do because various doctors may differ in their view regarding certain approaches of treatment that may not be clearly defined in the medical field. This is where implementation of the multidisciplinary care approach (discussed in Question 34) right from the time of diagnosis is advisable. It is a critical component of the medical care you should receive and may minimize your uncertainties regarding your cancer diagnosis and treatment. It is important, at least, to hear the opinion of different types of specialists. For example, the view of an oncologist about treatment of stage IV metastatic disease that has spread beyond the liver would be critical while you are still receiving local therapy, such as embolization (see Question 34) under the care of an interventional radiologist. On the other hand, patients should try to avoid getting too many opinions that may make things more confusing or even delay critical therapy. At the initial diagnosis, seeking a second opinion could be very valuable, because certain therapeutic options, such as surgery or liver transplantation, might not be available locally and a patient might need to seek medical care at a larger cancer center. In patients with very advanced disease, the need for a second opinion is less critical. Some patients and their families might take the challenge of traveling distances to seek opinions and look for miracles. In this instance, most doctors recommend using common sense and good judgment to determine the need for such second opinions. More importantly, you need to have a frank and open discussion with your physician, who is in the right position to assess the usefulness of a second opinion. Do not be surprised if your physician is the one who suggests a second opinion. In either instance, this is not a reflection on the inability of your physician to handle the current medical situation but is rather a genuine effort to make you feel comfortable with the treatment that you will choose.

31. How should I manage my emotions now that I have been diagnosed with liver cancer?

People differ in the way that they react to any adverse event in life. Some patients might be geared emotionally to handle their new diagnosis with liver cancer and react positively, but others might see themselves facing difficult times as they deal with new emotions, feelings, and stress. Patients are not expected to understand their illness or to identify priorities immediately.

Accepting the diagnosis of cancer might take a while, because patients have to deal first with their fear, denial, and anger. Patients fear cancer in general because of the unknown and the uncertainty that it carries. Cancer may cause you to question your sense of purpose in life. Patients are encouraged to discuss this fear with their doctors, because the more they learn about their disease, the more they will feel in control of the situation and know better how to deal with bad news. Patients might react with denial and anger, and it is better to circumvent those emotions as well. Patients might direct their anger against other people. It is a very delicate situation, especially if people close to the patient, such as family members, also are angry. Patients and their loved ones are encouraged to spell out their fears and angers and to realize that they are facing the same situation and they need each others' help.

Guilt might be present also, especially because some of the causes of liver cancer listed previously result from a person's lifestyle, such as using shared needles for

Accepting the diagnosis of cancer might take a while, because patients have to deal first with their fear, denial, and anger.

Depression

A sad state of mind characterized by feeling tired, with an inability to concentrate, an inability to sleep, a decreased appetite, guilt, and thoughts of death. Although it may be a psychiatric illness, it also may occur in patients facing a serious illness, such as primary liver cancer or other forms of cancer.

intravenous drug use and consuming alcohol. Guilt is normal and is best dealt with by accepting the current condition. Some patients might start building positively on the current situation. One patient, realizing the consequences of his previous use of intravenous drugs, is now a licensed counselor who helps others.

The other common emotion of a cancer patient is **depression**, which is again a normal and expected reaction to the acceptance of the new diagnosis of liver cancer. Patients should be aware of its signs and symptoms, because many of them can be confounded with those of the cancer itself, such as a loss of appetite and a decreased level of energy. Fatigue commonly is seen among patients with cancer who are depressed and may be misinterpreted as due to the cancer or its therapy. Nonetheless, even the subtle feeling of being depressed should be shared with the physician so that corrective action can be taken.

Patients are encouraged to have an open discussion with their caregivers and seek help for any concerning feelings. In many instances, professional help from a psychiatrist or even medications might be needed, and this should be accepted as an integral part of the healing process. Other services include the efforts of social workers, priests or ministers from various faiths, and patient representatives; these helpful persons are readily available in today's clinics and hospitals.

32. What insurance and financial concerns does a patient need to address after a diagnosis of liver cancer?

This is an important aspect of today's medical care. Health care is expensive, and patients with liver cancer might need to stop working, at least temporarily, thus affecting their insurance coverage. After being diagnosed with liver cancer, you need to start collecting information about the health coverage options that you have. Does the health insurance company provide only in-network coverage, thus making a patient select from the different providers and/or hospitals that his or her insurance company has an agreement with? Is there out-of-network coverage that allows a patient to seek medical care where he or she may wish? All individuals should make sure that all of their insurance premiums are paid and that all information is up to date. Patients should make sure to document all contacts with their insurance company. Organized and well-documented information might save a great deal of trouble later on. Most clinics and hospitals have a patient financial services department. It is important to establish contact with such a department to understand your rights and obligations.

Based on the severity of the illness or the extent of the treatment prescribed, patients might be required to take a sick leave or even be placed on disability. This can be done through a workplace or private insurance disability policy that may already be in place.The government also has many programs that may help you. These are divided into two distinct categories. Programs that are not based on income or financial means include Medicare for patients older than 65 years of age. Details about the program may be found on the official website: www.medicare.gov. Another is Social Security (www.ssa.gov) for patients older than 65 years of age and Social Security disability (www.ssa.gov/benefits/disability/) for disabled workers and their family based on disabled status and their prior contribution to the program. U.S. veterans also might seek veterans' benefit through the U.S. Department of Veterans Affairs (www.va.gov).

Health care is expensive, and patients with liver cancer might need to stop working, at least temporarily, thus affecting their insurance coverage.

If a patient does not have the means to obtain health care, he or she may seek government support through Medicaid. Details about the program can be found at www.medicaid.gov.

Similarly, you need to verify if you have a medication coverage plan. New cancer therapies and other supportive medications (e.g., antinausea medicines) are available in the form of pills. Some of the newer ones, called biologic therapies, are extremely expensive. Understanding your coverage plan and benefits early may give you a chance to identify and rectify any limiting issues, so your cancer therapy isn't delayed. Make sure to ask, as you may not necessarily be aware of all the resources that are available to you.

PART SIX

Treatment

Which treatment options are available for liver cancer?

What is multidisciplinary care?

What determines whether a tumor can be removed?

More . . .

33. Which treatment options are available for liver cancer?

Several treatment options are available for patients with HCC (**Box 4**). In general, the most effective therapy is to remove the tumor. This can be done in two ways. One method is to remove the part of the liver that contains the tumor. This is called **liver resection** or **partial hepatectomy**. The other option is to remove your entire liver and replace it with a new liver. This is called *liver transplantation*.

Liver resection

The surgical removal of all or a portion of the liver.

Partial hepatectomy

The surgical removal of part of the liver.

Ablation

The destruction of a tumor without actually removing it.

Alcohol injection

Inserting alcohol through a needle into a tumor. This technique is widely used to treat small hepatomas. Alcohol is directly toxic to the tumor.

Radiofrequency ablation

A form of tumor ablation that relies on heating to destroy tumor cells.

If the tumor cannot be removed, but is still limited to the liver, then your doctors may recommend an **ablation** procedure. There are several principal therapeutic procedures: **Alcohol injection** is performed by injecting alcohol directly into the tumor, which nowadays is less commonly used in view of the advent of other therapeutic options like **radiofrequency ablation** (also known as RFA), done by inserting a metal probe

Box 4 Treatments for Hepatocellular Cancer

Liver resection
Liver transplantation
Hepatic artery embolization
Radiofrequency ablation
Alcohol injection
Cryotherapy
Chemotherapy
Investigational chemotherapy
Biologic and targeted therapy
Supportive care
Investigational biologic or targeted therapy

into the tumor to heat it up in order to kill the cancer cells. **Cryotherapy** is performed with a metal probe that freezes the tumor. Hepatic artery embolization is a procedure in which the blood vessels of your tumor are clogged by injecting them with a substance; radioactive bead ablation is a procedure in which very small beads called microspheres containing radioactive material are injected into the blood vessels feeding your tumor to directly kill the tumor. Chemotherapy may be used in conjunction with **hepatic artery embolization**; this is referred to as **chemoembolization**. External beam radiation or radiotherapy is also now being evaluated but cannot be considered yet a standard of care.

Cryotherapy

A form of therapy that uses cold temperature to kill cancer cells.

You may not be a candidate for any of the above procedures because your tumor has not responded to them previously, your tumor has spread to too many sites within the liver, or your cancer has metastasized outside the liver. In any of these situations, systemic therapy is the appropriate treatment. Systemic therapy may consist of biologic therapy, immunotherapy chemotherapy, or both. These may be given either as pills, intravenously, or both. These drugs can travel almost anywhere in the body and attack the cancer wherever it may be. It may involve approved drugs or new agents that are under investigation. These treatments are discussed in detail later.

Hepatic artery embolization (chemoembolization)

The injection of microscopic particles (either attached to a chemotherapy drug or not) into the branches of the hepatic artery in order to ablate or destroy a liver tumor. The treatment works by blocking the blood supply to the tumor and, when chemotherapy is used, by delivering chemotherapy to the tumor.

34. What is multidisciplinary care?

Liver cancer is a very complex disease that requires the input of different specialists. Typically, you may have been followed by a hepatologist or gastroenterologist as part of a screening program because you are at risk for developing liver cancer (see Question 16) or because of other liver abnormalities. If liver cancer were to develop, it is advisable that your doctor presents your case at a multidisciplinary meeting or forum where doctors with interest in liver cancer who are from different specialties confer on a regular basis. The multidisciplinary team typically consists of surgeons, interventional radiologists, medical oncologists, hepatologists, and/or gastroenterologists. Other specialists may be present depending on what other services are offered at your medical facility. These may include transplant surgeons and radiation oncologists.

Hepatobiliary surgeon

A doctor who specializes in the surgical and ablative treatments of liver, gallbladder, bile duct, and pancreas tumors.

Surgeons and, more specifically, **hepatobiliary surgeons** who specialize in liver surgery, will decide whether your tumor can be removed. You may be referred to a liver transplant surgeon if liver transplantation is a consideration. Interventional radiologists specialize in delivering local ablative therapies. However, certain hepatobiliary and transplant surgeons may also perform radiofrequency ablation. A medical oncologist is a cancer doctor who specializes in the use of systemic therapy, which includes biologic therapy and chemotherapy. A hepatologist is a doctor who deals specifically with liver diseases, including cirrhosis and its complications.

Based on the extent of your cancer and the degree of cirrhosis, the choice of therapy is selected. In most instances the choice of therapy is straightforward. A single tumor in a normal or mildly cirrhotic liver is usually treated with surgical resection. If the liver cirrhosis is advanced, transplant would be contemplated if the number and size of the tumor(s) is within a predefined limit. For liver lesions that are not amenable to resection but are still limited to the liver, a local therapeutic procedure such as hepatic artery embolization may be warranted. In the case of HCC that has spread outside the liver, systemic therapy in the form of biologic and/or chemotherapy is necessary. You can imagine that not all medical situations would be straightforward and thus there is value to having a multidisciplinary team. Having your case discussed in this open format where specialists give their opinion about the best approach to treat your cancer will undoubtedly help you receive the most appropriate treatment. It is important to stress that physicians are used to this meeting format and are usually open to critique and different opinions. This approach emanates from their basic understanding of the complexity of the human body, diseases, and medicine, where there could be more than one answer to a problem. In the rare instance when you continue to receive a certain modality of treatment despite its inappropriateness, having your case presented at a multidisciplinary conference would be very valuable so your care can be redirected. Do not hesitate to ask or support your doctor to have your case presented at a multidisciplinary meeting or in a multidisciplinary forum.

Immediately after my father was diagnosed, the doctors recommended that he undergo resection to remove the single tumor in his liver. This course of action offered the best hope of a complete cure. His general health was very good, and the tumor was isolated in the left lobe of his liver. Much to our chagrin, though, the hepatobiliary surgeon decided, after closer investigation, that his liver was too cirrhotic and that recovery from resection would be too risky.

Therefore, over the next 4 years, his doctors focused on managing the tumor(s) by a combination of alcohol (ethanol) injections and embolizations. This regimen worked well for my father and preserved a good quality of life for him.

35. What determines whether a tumor can be removed?

Several factors determine whether a liver tumor can be removed. These include (1) the health of the patient, (2) the condition of the portion of your liver without the tumor, and (3) the distribution of the cancer and its relationship to vital structures of the liver. First, the patient must be in adequate general health in order to tolerate general **anesthesia** and a major operation such as liver resection. For instance, if a patient has a weak heart, an attempt at a liver resection may not be advisable because it may be too dangerous. The noncancerous part of your liver must be healthy enough in order to undergo a liver resection. The liver is a unique organ because it can grow again after part of it is removed. The liver is divided into right and left lobes, and it is composed of a total of eight individual segments. Up to six segments of a healthy liver can be removed in some patients. Remarkably, the liver regrows within 2 weeks after resection. Normal liver function is restored within 4 weeks of a liver resection. If the liver is healthy, up to about 80 percent of it can be removed safely. However, many patients with HCC have cirrhosis of the liver (discussed previously); thus, often only a small percentage of the liver can be safely removed. Most patients with advanced cirrhosis cannot undergo liver resection because they have a high chance of dying from the operation. They can die from bleeding that occurs during or shortly after the operation because patients with advanced cirrhosis may have varices or have difficulty in forming a blood clot. They also can die from liver failure in the first few weeks after liver resection. Their liver may function well enough for everyday living, but they may not be able to handle the stress of a liver resection.

Anesthesia

Medication that puts someone to sleep and/or reduces pain.

Several factors determine whether a liver tumor can be removed.

In some patients, the liver that will remain after operation is judged to be insufficient in size. Depending on the degree of cirrhosis and the amount of liver expected to be removed, your surgeon may elect to grow a portion of your liver prior to operation. This can be done using a procedure called portal vein embolization. Basically, an interventional radiologist injects a substance into the portal vein on the side of your tumor to decrease blood flow to that portion of your liver. This stimulates the other side of your liver to grow. In essence, the percentage of your liver that will then be removed is reduced, making it easier for you to recover from the planned operation.

Additional surgical factors relate to the extent of the cancer within the liver and its relationship to the vital structures of the liver. Most patients who are treated with liver resection have a single tumor. Sometimes, patients with two or three tumors also will be treated with liver resection. Patients with more than three tumors usually are not offered resection as an option because it is less beneficial in them, as the cancer may recur quickly. The vital structures of the liver include the bile duct, which carries bile out of the liver, and the blood vessels. Blood is brought into the liver via the **hepatic artery** and the **portal vein**. The bile duct, hepatic artery, and portal vein branch into left and right branches, which in turn branch many more times. Blood is removed from the liver via the three hepatic veins. A large vein, called the **inferior vena cava**, is behind the liver and gets blood from the hepatic veins and also directly from small branches from the liver that drain directly into it. The inferior vena cava also returns all of the blood from the lower half of your body to the heart. At the end of a liver resection, the patient must have at least one intact bile duct, portal vein, and hepatic artery branch and at least one hepatic vein (**Figure 2**).

Hepatic artery

The blood vessel that carries oxygenated blood to the liver.

Portal vein

A blood vessel that carries blood from the intestines to within the liver.

Inferior vena cava

A large vein that is supplied by multiple veins from the lower parts of the body and helps bring the blood back to the heart.

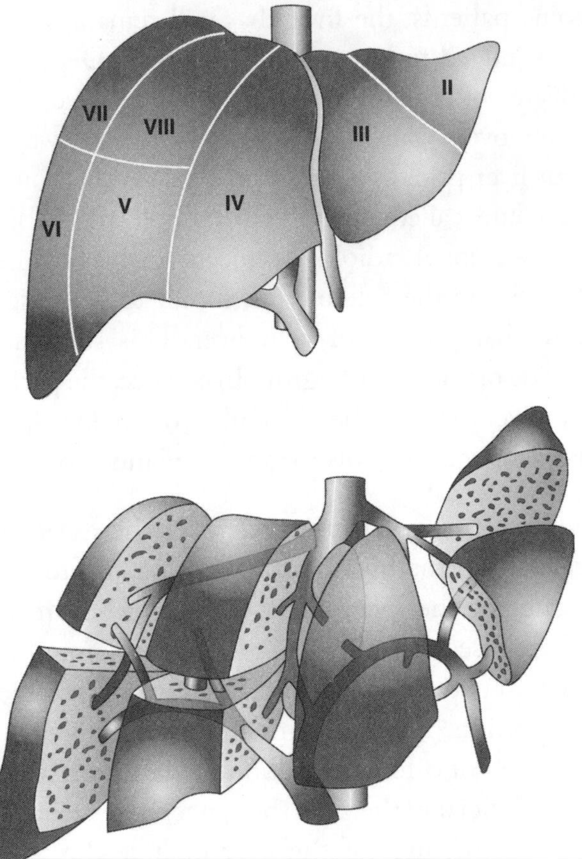

Figure 2 The liver is made up of eight segments, each with its own blood supply, blood drainage, and bile drainage.
Reprinted with permission of Memorial Sloan Kettering Cancer Center.

36. What preparations are made before a liver resection?

After the patient and doctor decide that a liver resection should be attempted, certain preparations will be made. If the patient is older or has certain medical problems, he or she may need to see a general medicine doctor or a cardiologist to determine whether he or she is fit enough for an operation. He or she may even be asked to undergo certain special tests. For instance, a patient may be given a stress test or **echocardiogram** to evaluate his or her heart function.

Next, the patient will get what is called preadmission testing. This includes routine blood tests, an **electrocardiogram**, and a chest x-ray. This is standard practice before undergoing general anesthesia. Often the patient will meet an **anesthesiologist**. In most cases, patients will be admitted the day of the operation. If special medical circumstances exist, a patient may be admitted to the hospital for 1 day or a few days before the operation. Depending on the location of the tumor, the surgeon may have the patient undergo a colon preparation using some medication to clean out the intestines before surgery.

On the morning of surgery, the patient is not allowed to eat or drink. The physician will have told you whether to take your normal medications with a sip of water. You will be asked to arrive at the hospital several hours before the scheduled time of the operation. You may be asked to arrive as early as 6 a.m. so everything is set in time before the surgery. Most surgeons start operating early in the morning. You will be asked to get undressed and to put on a hospital gown. Patients generally will be kept in a comfortable waiting area called the holding area until the operating room is ready. In some hospitals, families may be able to stay with the patient at that time. Several different people will likely ask you for your name, your medical history, the intended surgical procedure, and your allergies. Such repetition may become annoying, but it is done to ensure your safety.

Ultimately, the patient is taken into the operating room. This usually is done using a wheelchair. You will meet several nurses, surgical assistants, an anesthesiologist, and the surgeon. The operating room often is somewhat

Echocardiogram

A test for the heart in which pictures and functional values of the heart are obtained using ultrasound.

Electrocardiogram

An electrical tracing of the heart.

Anesthesiologist

A doctor who specializes in the delivery of anesthesia.

cold, but you will be covered with several blankets during the operation. An intravenous (IV) drip will be started in your arm if it was not placed already in the holding area. You will be placed flat on a table and asked to breathe through a mask and then will be put to sleep.

37. What happens during a liver resection?

After you are asleep, the hair (if you have any) that is on your belly will be shaved, and your belly will be washed with soap. Generally, a small tube, called a **Foley catheter**, will be placed into the bladder so that the amount of urine can be closely monitored. A larger IV may be placed into your neck to give additional fluids and/or medications that might be needed for support through the operation.

Foley catheter

A tube that is placed into the bladder to monitor precisely the urine output of a patient.

In some circumstances, the surgeon may decide to perform a **laparoscopy** immediately before your liver resection or sometime beforehand. A laparoscopy is performed with the patient under general anesthesia. A few small incisions (less than an inch) are made in order to insert a telescope and some instruments in order to inspect the belly. Specifically, the surgeon is looking to see whether the cancer is more advanced or has spread outside of the liver, which sometimes cannot be seen on the radiologic tests that were done before surgery. If you have cirrhosis, the surgeon also determines whether your cirrhosis is too advanced for you to undergo an operation safely.

Laparoscopy

A procedure that is done under general anesthesia and performed by a surgeon in which the inside of the abdomen can be examined through a few small incisions.

The surgeon may decide to perform the liver resection using laparoscopy. Alternatively, a number of different incisions can be made to expose the liver during an

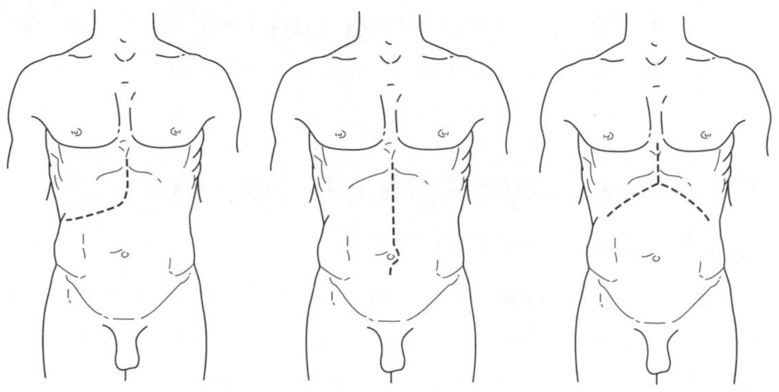

Figure 3 The three most common incisions for liver surgery are shown by the dotted lines.

Reprinted with permission of Memorial Sloan Kettering Cancer Center.

open operation. The three most common are shown in **Figure 3**. Your surgeon will determine whether your tumor can be removed. Although your tumor may appear to be removable on a CT scan or MRI, the surgeon may find that your tumor cannot be removed because of any one of several findings:

1. The tumor has spread to the outside of the liver.
2. The tumor has spread to other areas within your liver.
3. The tumor cannot be safely removed from vital structures.
4. There is more advanced cirrhosis than anticipated.

If the tumor is removable, the surgeon then will proceed with liver resection. As part of the operation, the surgeon may have to remove your gallbladder to expose other structures of the liver. The gallbladder is a small organ that is situated on the edge of your liver and functions as a storage tank for bile. Bile is stored in the gallbladder and is emptied into the intestine after we eat a meal. It helps you digest a large fatty meal. Patients can live a perfectly normal life without a gallbladder.

38. What happens in the hospital after a liver resection?

After the operation, you will be taken to a recovery room for close observation. The main risk within the first 12 hours is bleeding from the cut surface of the liver. Rarely, a patient needs to undergo an emergency operation to control bleeding. Depending on the hospital, you will stay in a highly monitored setting for 1 to 5 days and then be transferred to a regular patient floor. Overall, you can expect to be in the hospital between 2 and 10 days depending on whether the operation was performed laparoscopically or not, the size of the liver resection, and your general health. If everything goes well, you should be able to sit in a chair and in many cases, walk the day after your surgery. It often takes a few days before you are ready to eat again. A special intravenous pump that you control provides pain medication or you may have an epidural that delivers pain medication directly near your spinal cord. The nurse will explain how to use it.

39. What are the risks of a liver resection?

Other potential complications of liver resection exist besides bleeding. Many patients will temporarily gain weight from the extra fluids that are given around the time of the operation. You may notice that your ankles are swollen from this. In some patients, the incision may not heal completely and actually separate slightly. This will require dressing changes while you are in the hospital and perhaps also when you are at home. About 10 percent of the time, a fluid collection will form where the liver was removed, and it will require drainage about a week later. This is usually done by having an **interventional radiologist** insert a needle or a small drain into the collection. Other complications include **pneumonia** or infection in your urine because of the temporary tube that was placed into the bladder.

Patients with cirrhosis are at an additional risk of complications from an operation. They may develop gastrointestinal bleeding, which may arise from **gastritis** (stomach irritation), an **ulcer**, or **varices**. Varices are dilated veins in the esophagus or stomach. The veins dilate because the pressure within a cirrhotic liver is higher than normal. Patients with cirrhosis also are at risk for ascites, which is the accumulation of fluid within the belly. Ascites is generally treated with **diuretics (water pills)** that make you urinate more frequently.

Occasionally, a patient will die after a liver resection because the remaining liver fails. Heart attack and stroke are other potential complications.

After you go home, complete recovery will take place over the next 3 to 6 weeks. You will slowly regain your energy. You may not notice that you are improving each day, but each week you will likely feel better. If you are not, then you should notify your doctor. Usually, if your doctor agrees, you can drive in a few weeks. You should be totally off pain medications by then. You should not do any heavy lifting for several months so that you do not disrupt the incision. You should generally expect to regain your quality of life, although your doctor can discuss specific concerns related to your condition.

Interventional radiologist

A doctor who specializes in performing procedures under radiologic (ultrasound, x-ray, or CT scan) guidance such as tumor biopsies, hepatic artery embolization, or a mediport.

Pneumonia

A lung infection.

Gastritis

Inflammation of the inside lining of the stomach.

Ulcer

A lesion of the stomach that results from inflammation and may bleed.

Varix

An abnormally swollen vein that is prone to bleed.

Diuretics (water pills)

Drugs that increase the discharge of urine.

40. What is included in the pathology report from my surgery?

The pathology report from your liver resection contains a lot of information. From it, the precise stage of the cancer can be determined. The written report will state the size and number of the tumors. If lymph nodes were removed, the report will state whether tumor cells existed in them. Unlike many other cancers that are removed, in HCC, surgeons generally remove only the lymph nodes around the liver if they think that the nodes contain cancer. This is because most patients undergoing liver resections for HCC do not have involved nodes. Also, most surgeons will not remove the liver if lymph nodes are involved because, in general, the benefit of the operation is less because the chance of the cancer recurring is higher. The pathologist determines whether the surgeon achieved a negative margin of resection by entirely removing the tumor with a rim of normal tissue as a margin. The pathologist also dissects the liver and looks at the tumor under the microscope to determine whether the tumor invaded any large or small blood vessels. Patients with vascular invasion have a higher rate of having their tumor come back in the future. The other piece of information is the status of the noncancerous liver. The pathologist will determine whether the liver has any signs of damage or cirrhosis. If so, the pathologist will give a grade for the degree of cirrhosis present.

After you go home, complete recovery will take place over the next 3 to 6 weeks.

41. Will I be cured after a liver resection?

In general, no one can predict whether your liver tumor will come back after it is removed. Some patients are truly cured, meaning that their tumor never returns.

Many patients, however, will have their tumor return at some point. If you have liver cirrhosis, you also are at risk of developing a new tumor. This happens for the same reasons that led to your original tumor. Thus, you should be followed carefully after your liver operation. If your blood level of AFP was elevated before the operation, then it is a good marker of whether your tumor has come back. It should be measured two to three times per year. The other primary method of surveillance after an operation is a CT, an MRI, or an ultrasound of your abdomen. These are often done two to four times per year for the first few years.

Doctors normally measure the outcome of patients with cancer by determining what percentage will be alive at 5 years. Again, it is important to stress that doctors generally cannot reliably predict what will happen to any given patient. It is like grades in school. The average grade in a class may be a "C"; however, some patients do a lot better, and others do a lot worse. The likelihood of survival at 5 years depends on a number of factors, including the size and number of the tumors, the health of your uninvolved liver, and your general medical condition. Your doctors will counsel you about your likely outcome.

42. Should I receive adjuvant therapy after a liver resection to prevent a recurrence of the tumor?

Adjuvant therapy is the use of chemotherapy, biologic therapy, immunotherapy, radiation, or any other form of treatment that is given after a cancer is surgically removed. In some other types of cancer, chemotherapy routinely is given after the surgical removal of the tumor. It is done in an effort to kill any few cells of cancer

Adjuvant therapy

A form of therapy that will help prevent the recurrence of cancer after a potentially curative treatment such as surgery.

that might remain and thus helps to prevent the recurrence of the cancer. However, at this time, the standard of care after the removal of hepatocellular carcinoma is simply to observe the patient. Several clinical trials of adjuvant therapy suggested its benefit after the removal of a HCC; however, although promising, the results of these clinical trials were never reproduced, making the true value of these approaches uncertain. Other postoperative treatment, including sorafenib (Nexavar®) therapy, was evaluated but did not show any added benefit as adjuvant therapy after surgical resection or ablation. It is discussed in Question 43 as a suppressor of the hepatitis virus, which is a cause of the cancer.

Clinical trial

A research study that answers many of the questions regarding newly discovered therapies.

Currently, other **clinical trials** are evaluating different therapies, including immunotherapy. Until this clinical trial is complete and its results are reported, any adjuvant therapy outside of this clinical trial is not recommended. You can of course always check on trials that are available, as well as their status, at www.clinicaltrials.gov.

43. If the tumor cannot be resected now, can I have therapy first and then go to surgery?

Neoadjuvant treatment

Therapy that is given before surgical removal of a cancer, aiming at reducing its size and rendering it more resectable.

Therapy including chemotherapy, biologic therapy, or immunotherapy that is given before surgery in order to shrink the tumor and to allow it to be resected is called neoadjuvant therapy. As with adjuvant therapy, no established standard of care is available for **neoadjuvant treatment**. The best data come from a limited study that was performed at the Chinese University of Hong Kong where 50 patients were tried on a combination of three chemotherapy drugs (cisplatin, doxorubicin, and 5-fluorouracil) and interferon (an immune booster) known as PIAF (see Question 70). Of the 50 patients, 13 had a major response to therapy, and of the 13, 9 went back to surgery and had their tumor resected. Out of the 9, 4 patients had no tumor left behind in their removed part of the liver. Although this approach is not established as a standard of care, it can undoubtedly be used if it seems feasible based on a discussion among the patient, surgeon, and medical oncologist.

44. What happens if my tumor comes back?

Your doctor may discover that your tumor has come back based on new symptoms or radiologic tests, which may be supported by the serum AFP level. Several options are available if your tumor returns. Approximately 10 percent of the time, you may be eligible for another liver resection. Reoperation depends on the same factors listed in Question 35 and the extent of the first liver operation. The other treatment options include all of those listed later here for initially unresectable tumors—liver transplantation, tumor ablation, biologic therapy, chemotherapy, clinical trials, or supportive care.

45. Why is liver transplantation performed for liver cancer? When is it performed?

Liver transplantation is recommended sometimes for patients with hepatocellular carcinoma for several reasons. First, the entire liver is removed as part of liver transplantation. This removes the tumor as well as any single cells that may have spread from the tumor to other areas of the liver; these may not be taken care of by a regular surgical resection that gets rid of only the tumors seen to the naked eye of the surgeon. These microscopic cells, if present, may result in tumor recurrence if just part of the liver were removed. In fact, in the vast majority of patients whose tumor comes back, it recurs initially in the remaining portion of the liver. The other major rationale to remove the entire liver exists for patients with cirrhosis. The new liver will have normal function; thus, the patient will no longer be at risk for the complications of cirrhosis. Nevertheless, viral hepatitis infection may recur in the new liver, and continued excessive alcohol use may affect the function of the new liver.

Various guidelines exist that state which patients with liver cancer should receive a liver transplant. The most widely used are as follows: a single tumor that is less than 5 cm or three tumors that are each less than 3 cm, no evidence of blood vessel invasion on radiologic studies, and no evidence of cancer that has spread outside the liver. Tumor invasion of blood vessels identifies patients who are at high risk for having the tumor spread to other areas of their body, and patients with blood vessel invasion, as well as those with tumors larger than 5 cm or with many tumors, may have less benefit from a liver transplantation. Other considerations, such as patient age, exist. Patients over 70 years old are less likely to be considered candidates for transplantation. Other factors that may make you ineligible for a liver transplant are severe heart or lung disease, active alcohol abuse, prior cancer, active infection, or a psychiatric condition that may interfere with your ability to comply with medical care.

It is important to know that a proper clinical trial has never been performed to determine whether liver resection or liver transplantation is better. Such a trial would be difficult to conduct, because patients would have to consent to receiving one of the two treatments in a randomized way (e.g., by tossing a coin). From a number of published series of liver resection and transplantation, the survival appears similar between the two treatments, although this topic is highly controversial among surgeons.

Because my father had recovered successfully from an unrelated colon cancer over a decade ago, this made him an unlikely (low priority) organ candidate. We were advised that liver transplantation was not appropriate for him. The major problems with liver transplantation, from a caregiver's point of view, are not only the long waiting period, but also deciding when to pursue a liver transplant as the first option.

It is important to know that a proper clinical trial has never been performed to determine whether liver resection or liver transplantation is better.

46. From where do new livers come?

A new liver may come from one of two sources: a cadaver or a living donor. A cadaveric liver is obtained from a person whose brain has died but his or her organs are still alive. For instance, a person may die in an automobile accident, but his or her organs remain functional for a short period of time thereafter. The organs are donated for transplantation if the family agrees or the donor had decided this. An international organization called the United Network for Organ Sharing (UNOS) distributes the available organs to patients on the transplant waiting list. Patients are given organs based on their degree of liver function and whether they have biological similarities with the donor (blood type and body size). The waiting time for a liver is variable but could be as long as a few years because there is a shortage of donor livers compared with the number of patients who need liver transplants.

MELD (Model for End-Stage Liver Disease)

A mathematical equation that is used to prioritize patients for liver transplantation based on their laboratory values.

Creatinine

A substance usually excreted from the body through urine. It is used to help assess kidney function.

Bilirubin

A component of bile that comes from the breakdown of red blood cells.

Prothrombin

A protein produced by the liver that helps blood to clot.

UNOS prioritizes patients to receive a cadaveric liver with a scoring system. The **MELD (Model for End-Stage Liver Disease)** is a score that is based on your blood work. Specifically, your **creatinine** (which reflects kidney function), and **bilirubin** and **prothrombin** time (both reflect liver function) determine your score. The score ranges from 6 to 40. The higher your score is, the more likely that you will receive a liver. Patients with cancer are given an additional number of points. Otherwise, many of them would never get an organ because there are many patients in full liver failure without cancer who would get priority.

The other source of a new liver is from a living donor: A family member or friend agrees to donate part of their liver. In many cases, this may significantly extend the patient's life and prevent the patient from dying while on a waiting list for a cadaveric liver. Every effort is made to minimize potential complications to the donor. However, liver resection is a major operation. Rarely, people have died donating their liver to someone else.

To give you an idea of how liver transplantation is used for HCC, close to 6,000 liver transplants are performed in the United States each year, of which less than 300 are from living donors. Only about 5 to 10 percent of transplants are performed for HCC.

47. How am I evaluated for a liver transplant?

Human immunodeficiency virus (HIV)

A virus that destroys helper cells of the immune system that usually fight infections and may lead to AIDS.

Liver transplantation is carried out at specialized centers. The evaluation process is quite extensive, because liver transplantation is such a large operation and donor livers are scarce. You will undergo extensive blood testing. In particular, you will be tested for previous hepatitis infection and **human immunodeficiency virus (HIV)**, the virus that is responsible for AIDS. You will have several radiologic tests that may include a CT scan, an MRI, an ultrasound, an **endoscopy** to determine whether you have varices (see Question 39), and **arteriography** to look at your blood vessels. The remainder of the evaluation will be like that described for liver resection.

Endoscopy

A procedure performed by a gastroenterologist. A tube is placed into your mouth while you are lightly sedated. The doctor can then look at the inside of the stomach and the first part of the intestine to search for dilated blood vessels (varices), ulcers, or gastritis.

Numerous types of doctors and associated healthcare personnel who work together will determine whether you are a suitable candidate for a liver transplant. These include a transplant surgeon, a hepatologist, a transplant coordinator who will work with you closely before and after a transplant, a social worker, and a psychologist or a psychiatrist who will help you and your family manage the psychologic stress of undergoing a transplant.

Arteriography

A radiologic test that demonstrates the artery branches of a person. The technique is performed by an interventional radiologist. Typically, a small tube is inserted into the patient's leg during the procedure. A contrast agent is injected, and x-rays are then taken to reveal the arteries.

48. What will happen while I am on the waiting list?

If you are placed on a transplant waiting list for a cadaveric liver, you will be evaluated periodically to assess your liver function and the extent of your tumor. While you are waiting, your doctors may want to treat your cancer and may recommend a localized procedure, including hepatic artery embolization, alcohol injection, radiofrequency ablation, or less commonly, a surgical resection.

You will be monitored regularly (e.g., every 3 months) to determine the extent of your tumor. You do run the risk of your tumor progressing to the point that you are no longer eligible for transplantation. While waiting, some patients actually die because of liver failure or tumor progression. You may no longer be eligible for a transplant if your tumor progresses because you may no longer fulfill the criteria for a transplant (see Question 45). In other words, if your tumor becomes extensive, a transplant may no longer help you.

You do run the risk of your tumor progressing to the point that you are no longer eligible for transplantation.

49. What is involved in a cadaveric liver transplant?

You will be notified immediately if a cadaver liver organ becomes available and you will be rushed into the hospital and prepared for surgery. Occasionally, the donor liver will be found to be inadequate or not suitable for you, and the intended transplant will be aborted. You will then go back on the waiting list. If the organ is suitable, you then will undergo a 4- to 8-hour operation to remove your existing liver and to implant the new liver. After the operation, you will be placed in the intensive care unit for a few days while you are recovering. You will have multiple tubes in your body to help your doctors take better care of you and your blood work will be monitored very closely. You can expect to spend 1 to 2 weeks in the hospital recovering. During this time, you will be taught about the new medications that you must take to reduce your immune function so that your body does not reject your new liver.

50. What is involved in a living related donor liver transplantation?

If you receive a living related donor liver, you and the donor generally will be admitted the morning of surgery. The donor operation will take about 3 to 4 hours, and the donor will be in the hospital for about 5 to 7 days. You will be given part of the donor's liver. The newly transplanted part will undergo regeneration in your body to provide you with a normal-sized liver. The donor's remaining liver also must regenerate.

Certainly, there are potential psychologic implications for both the donor and the recipient. Sometimes the donor may feel that he or she has no choice in undergoing the operation to donate part of his or her liver. Pressure from the family, friends, or the patient may be responsible for this. Conversely, the recipient may experience guilt for putting the donor through a partial hepatectomy, especially if the donor suffers a complication. The transplant team typically includes a psychologist/psychiatrist who will help address these issues. It is normal to ask such professionals for advice during the transplantation evaluation or after surgery.

51. What are the complications of liver transplantation?

Because of the technical complexity of performing a liver transplant and the immunologic aspects of receiving a new liver, several potential complications exist after liver transplantation:

1. Bleeding: Just as with liver resection, occasionally a patient must undergo another operation for bleeding shortly after the original operation.
2. Hepatic artery clotting or **thrombosis**: Sometimes, the hepatic artery, which is one of the blood vessels that supplies the liver with fresh blood, can clot. Another operation may be needed to address this problem. In the worst case, another liver transplant may have to be performed.
3. Primary liver nonfunction: In some patients, the new liver fails to work properly for unexplained reasons. Another liver may have to be transplanted immediately.
4. Biliary leak: In some patients, bile can leak from the connection of the old bile duct to the new bile duct. This usually resolves with conservative therapy.

Thrombosis

The formation of clots.

5. Infection: Infection can occur at anytime after transplantation because you will be taking medication that suppresses your **immune system**. You will be taught that any sign of infection requires immediate medical attention because otherwise, even with a minor infection, your life could be threatened.

Immune system

An intricate body system that protects people against foreign organisms or toxins that may cause disease.

6. Rejection: Your body may try to reject your new liver. Generally, **rejection** can be stopped by altering the immune-suppressing drugs that you are taking. A liver biopsy performed by placing a needle in your side may be performed to diagnose the extent of the rejection. It is very important to take your medications and to comply with frequent medical monitoring to avoid rejection.

Rejection

The process by which the body refuses a donated transplanted liver and regards it as foreign.

7. Recurrent hepatitis: Most patients with chronic hepatitis B or C will have recurrence of hepatitis in the new liver. The concern is that the virus is still circulating in the blood of a patient previously infected with hepatitis and can relocate and attack the new liver, thus causing hepatitis.

52. Will I be cured after a liver transplantation? Can I prevent the cancer from returning after transplantation?

Overall, liver transplantation is safe and highly successful. In patients without liver cancer, the 1-year survival is approximately 90 percent, and the 5-year survival is approximately 80 percent. In patients with liver cancer, survival is determined mostly by whether the tumor comes back. The 5-year survival is generally between

50 percent and 75 percent. The resumption of a normal quality of life is expected.

53. Can I suppress the hepatitis from recurring and infecting the new liver?

Using antiviral therapy (see Questions 9 and 10) to suppress virus replication, one might hope to reduce the damage to the liver cells and thus decrease the risk of developing cancer again. New hepatitis C antivirus therapies have been shown to be effective after transplant. Your doctor will discuss this option with you.

54. What is tumor ablation?

Ablation is the destruction of a tumor without actually removing it. In some cases, the entire tumor can be destroyed, especially if the tumor is less than 3 cm in diameter. With larger tumors, it is more likely that a small part of the tumor will survive and begin to grow again at some point. Several techniques of ablation exist; hepatic artery embolization (with or without chemotherapy), radioembolization, radio-frequency ablation, and cryotherapy are the most widely used. Each method acts in a different way, as described later. Some physicians will use them in combination. For instance, an embolization can be performed followed by radiofrequency ablation. Any of the various procedures can be repeated in the future if your tumor grows back. If you have multiple or large tumors, your doctors may elect to apply those procedures a few times within the first 2 months of diagnosis, in order to treat all of your cancer. However, your multidisciplinary team needs to discuss this to ensure that only appropriate therapy is considered; other beneficial therapies, such as chemotherapy, are discussed as well.

55. What is hepatic artery embolization?

Hepatic artery embolization is the injection of particles into the hepatic artery in order to destroy the tumor. The particles can be considered as "microscopic sand" that clogs the blood vessels feeding the tumor. Hepatocellular carcinoma depends largely on blood supplied by the hepatic artery to survive. Part of the hepatic artery can be clogged because your liver receives blood from another vessel called the portal vein. Many doctors inject chemotherapy or use particles called drug eluting beads, that have a chemotherapy agent attached to them. The authors and other members of the team at Memorial Sloan Kettering Cancer Center in a clinical trial found that chemotherapy does not add value and may add toxicity and thus recommend embolization without chemotherapy, known as bland embolization. Despite these findings, embolization with chemotherapy, also called chemoembolization, is still widely used worldwide.

A particular type of radiologist called an interventional radiologist performs hepatic artery embolization. These radiologists are specialized in performing invasive procedures under x-ray technology guidance. Usually, you come into the hospital on the day of the procedure. The procedure takes about 2 hours and you will be lightly sedated. The procedure is carried out while you are lying flat on a table. The skin in your leg (usually the right leg) is numbed with a tiny injection, then a small tube is placed into the main artery in your leg. An x-ray machine is positioned above you and is used to monitor the location of the small tube, which is passed through a large artery called the **aorta** and then into the hepatic artery, which feeds your liver. The tube is advanced into either

Aorta

The largest artery in the body. It originates from the heart, and its branches supply the entire body with blood containing oxygen.

the right or left branch of the hepatic artery. From there, particles can be released. In general, it is more desirable to occlude selectively the specific blood vessels that are supplying a tumor and to preserve the vessels going to a normal liver. At the end of the procedure, the small tube is removed from your leg. You will have to lay flat for 4 to 6 hours afterward to make sure that the wound heals and does not bleed.

Embolization can cause a number of side effects; thus, some patients are admitted to the hospital for a day or two. In general, the magnitude of the side effects is proportional to the amount of tumor that is destroyed. If you have a large tumor, you can expect to have a number of side effects if it was completely embolized because of the amount of dead tissue that results from the embolization. Dead tissue releases a lot of toxic substances into your bloodstream; these toxins can make you sick. The most common side effect is nausea. This can be controlled with special medication, but you may not wish to eat for a day or so. Pain can occur, and you will receive pain medication for relief. In the time period following the embolization, you may have a fever, and your doctors may notice an increase in some of the blood levels of liver enzymes. All of these side effects are collectively called post-embolization syndrome and should resolve with a few days to several weeks. Rarely, embolization will cause a problem with your heart or kidney function. Another unusual complication is the formation of an infection in the dead tumor tissue. This is called an **abscess**, which is treated with **antibiotics**. In rare situations, you may need a drain placed into the infection. Also, the tube that was placed into the artery may cause complications. Bleeding can occur at the puncture site and form a large bruise called a **hematoma** or pseudoaneurysm. Occasionally, a patient may require an

Abscess
A collection of pus.

Antibiotics
Medications used to fight infections.

Hematoma
A collection of blood.

Embolization can cause a number of side effects; thus, some patients are admitted to the hospital for a day or two.

operation to repair the blood vessel if it was damaged. The addition of chemotherapy to the embolization, also called chemoembolization, will of course add potential side effects from the chemotherapy.

56. Can I receive systemic therapy with embolization?

Since sorafenib is effective in advanced HCC, investigators studied whether it can improve the results of hepatic artery chemoembolization in unresectable HCC. Multiple clinical trials have been completed and none has shown any value for adding sorafenib to embolization; thus this is not recommended. Efforts evaluating the addition of immunotherapy to local therapies are underway based on scientific arguments that manipulation of the immune system by chemoembolization may be circumvented by the addition of immunotherapy. You can check if you are eligible for any of those trials at www.clinicaltrials.gov.

An argument that embolization will be valuable therapy to control the cancer in the liver despite the presence of spread out metastatic disease, which can be controlled with systemic therapy, is generally not recommended.

57. What is radiofrequency ablation and cryotherapy?

Radiofrequency ablation and cryotherapy are used to destroy a tumor by inserting a metal probe into the tumor and exposing it to extremes of temperature. Radiofrequency ablation heats the tumor, whereas cryotherapy freezes it. Radiofrequency ablation and cryotherapy can be used only if you have a limited number of tumors (usually less than five or six) that are small to medium in size (less than 3 cm), and can be used instead of surgery as a curative therapy. Either procedure can be performed in a variety of ways. An interventional radiologist can place the probe percutaneously (meaning through the skin), in which case sedation will be required during the procedure. Radiofrequency ablation and cryotherapy also can be performed via laparoscopy or during an open surgical operation. Both require general anesthesia. Laparoscopy involves several small incisions in your abdomen. Open laparotomy is performed through a cut in your belly. Your doctor will decide which access you require based on the number, size, and location of your tumors. For instance, not all liver tumors can be reached via the percutaneous approach. It is important to know that not all tumors can be treated with radiofrequency ablation or cryotherapy. If a tumor is close to a main bile duct, the use of these techniques may be too risky. If a tumor is near a large blood vessel, radiofrequency ablation and cryotherapy may not be advisable either. Some newer techniques for direct ablation, such as microwave ablation or adding chemotherapy to enhance radio-frequency ablation, are currently under study.

58. What is alcohol injection?

Exposure to pure alcohol directly can kill cells. Many patients with hepatocellular carcinoma have firm or hard livers because of their cirrhosis. In contrast, HCC is typically quite soft. When alcohol is injected directly into a tumor, the tumor soaks it up, whereas the surrounding firm liver does not. This is the basis for using an alcohol injection. Alcohol injection normally is performed percutaneously. Just as with radiofrequency ablation and cryotherapy, the number, size, and location of your tumors are important in determining whether alcohol injection can be performed. The treatment is administered by an interventional oncologist who guides a needle while the patient is under anesthesia. This procedure is now used very often, as radiofrequency ablation was shown to be more beneficial. Nonetheless it may be used in rare instances, especially because of technical limitation reasons that will prohibit the use of radiofrequency ablation.

59. What are biologic and targeted therapies?

Nowadays, scientists have come to a better understanding of how cancer cells keep producing. Scientists now know of specific steps in the cell reproduction that lead to this uncontrolled replication of cells, which causes cancer. They also have identified specific therapies that stop tumor replication or disrupt its blood supply. These new therapies and their targets operate like a key and a lock. While some therapies or keys are specific to certain targets or locks, others may have an effect on different targets like a master key. Similar to many other cancers, these new "targeted" or "biologic" therapies might play a role in primary liver cancer. They are also called tyrosine kinase inhibitors.

Many of them were and are being tested in different clinical trials. Sorafenib (Nexavar®), was the first to be approved by the Food and Drug Administration for use in the United States and by similar regulatory agencies in other parts of the world for the treatment of unresectable primary liver cancer. Other targeted or biologic drugs more recently have shown to be beneficial to patients with unresectable primary liver cancer. These include lenvatinib (Lenvima®), regorafenib (Stivarga®), and cabozantinib (Cabometyx®) which are already FDA approved; and ramicirumab (Cyramza®) that is yet to be approved. Sorafenib (Nexavar®) and lenvatinib (Lenvima®) both have been shown to be beneficial as a first systemic treatment for unresectable primary liver cancer. Your doctor would recommend regorafenib (Stivarga®) if you previously received sorafenib (Nexavar®), tolerated it, but now the cancer is not responding to it anymore. Cabozantinib (Cabometyx®) is indicated as second line or third line treatment. Pending approval, you may be prescribed ramicirumab (Cyramza®) as second line treatment if your alpha-fetoprotein (AFP) level is high and more than 400. Your doctor may prescribe any of these drugs if your primary liver cancer has spread outside of the liver, and in certain instances where the cancer is still limited to the liver but cannot be taken out surgically. None will cure your cancer. The aim of the treatment is to control the tumor, preventing it from spreading further. This means increasing your lifespan while having the cancer, which is called improved survival.

How to choose one of these different therapies remains unclear. Your doctor will use his/her experience and continuously emerging data to help guide you in your decision.

60. What are the side effects of the biologic and targeted therapies?

Although doctors call them targeted therapies, they are not as specific as one might think; thus, they can have side effects. Sorafenib and regorafenib might cause a rash over the palms and soles of the feet (also called hand-foot skin reaction), diarrhea, and fatigue, among other side effects. Hand-foot skin reaction is the most common of those toxicities and can be the most distressing if not handled appropriately. There are well-defined, established steps to help prevent and treat it. Those preventive and therapeutic approaches involve both you and your physician. Hand-foot skin reaction is graded 1 to 3 based on its intensity. Grade 1 indicates the fewest signs and symptoms. You might notice some redness over the fingers, toes, palms of your hands, or soles of your feet. There might be some painless swelling, numbness, or tingling. This discomfort generally would not interfere with your daily activities. Grade 2 implies the presence of painful redness and swelling. This would definitely interfere with daily activities such as buttoning your shirt or typing on your computer. Grade 3 will prevent you from performing daily activities. Symptoms include moist peeling of the skin, ulceration, blistering, and severe pain.

The aim of the treatment is. . . increasing your lifespan while having the cancer, called improved survival.

The most critical component of treating hand-foot skin reaction is prevention. Your doctor might ask you to see a podiatrist to remove old calluses or dead skin areas before starting treatment, as these are prone to develop hand-foot skin reaction. It is also important to avoid all irritants that might cause or worsen hand-foot skin reaction. Irritants include hot water, direct sunlight, tight footwear, excessive friction, vigorous activity, and contact with cleaning products containing strong chemicals. A critical step in this preventive approach is to keep your doctor informed about appearance of any of the symptoms or signs described above, or those that you find to be concerning. While your doctor will see you frequently, symptoms may occur in between visits. Be sure to contact your doctor as soon as possible.

Do your best to describe what your hands and feet look like, and make sure to report any pain and/or limitation of daily activities. An easy way to share this information, if your doctors approve it, is to send digital photographs using your mobile phone or digital camera and e-mail them to the doctor's office. The authors of this book have used this approach at Memorial Sloan Kettering Cancer Center, and it has proven very valuable in early prevention and intervention of hand-foot skin reaction. The pictures can also be compared over time to assess improvement or worsening of the condition. Based on the grade or extent of your symptoms, your doctor may recommend that you apply different moisturizing creams or cold packs, or he or she may prescribe pain medications. Your doctor may also suggest that you continue taking sorafenib or regorafenib at the same dose, at a lower dose, or that you stop taking it for a short period of time before resuming it at a lower dose. In rare instances, your doctor may decide to stop giving you sorafenib or regorafenib indefinitely.

Diarrhea generally is not severe, but close to 10 percent of patients may have close to seven bowel movements per day. Avoiding greasy or fried foods may help to prevent diarrhea. Typically, it starts 2 to 5 days after starting sorafenib. Your doctor may prescribe antidiarrheal medicine and may consider a reduction in the dose of sorafenib. Of note, constipation may also occur.

Fatigue can be difficult to appreciate or assess, as you may already feel tired because of the cancer and cirrhosis, and patients perceive fatigue differently. Your doctor may use a numeric rating scale or assessment tools to help better define the extent of your fatigue. As fatigue can be due to many factors, it is necessary to identify and treat all contributing factors, such as pain and poor nutrition. Exercise can reduce fatigue by increasing functional capacity. Good sleep patterns and avoiding long daytime naps so you can sleep better at night may also help. About 10 percent of patients may have enough fatigue to limit their daily activity and may require a reduction in the dose of sorafenib or regorafenib.

Another side effect of sorafenib or regorafenib is increased blood pressure, which may require starting or adding more blood pressure medications. Avoiding salt is always helpful, and it may also help your liver condition and reduce fluid accumulation in the abdomen and legs (see Question 86). Other rare side effects include mild hair thinning but very rarely hair loss, rash, itching, dry skin, reduced appetite, weight loss, abdominal pain, nausea, and vomiting.

Serious but rare side effects include blood in the stools or vomit. Bleeding may also occur in other sites of the body. Although this is very rare, it should be taken seriously and requires immediate emergency medical attention. Heart attacks, delayed or complicated healing of surgical or any other wounds, and perforation of the guts may also occur in rare instances.

It is important to note that if you have tolerated sorafenib and you are now taking regorafenib, you are more likely to tolerate it as well.

The most common side effect of lenvatinib is increased blood pressure, which can be managed like sorafenib and regorafenib. Fatigue, diarrhea, decreased appetite and possible decreased weight, joint pains, abdominal pain, and hand-foot skin reaction are less common but can possibly happen. Cabozantinib, similar to the other biologic and targeted therapies, can cause hand-foot skin reaction, fatigue, decreased appetite, diarrhea, and nausea. Ramicirumab side effects include hypertension, fatigue, alteration of liver function, and low platelets.

As for any other drug, side effects may be revised and new ones may be described. It is always recommended to refer to the package insert of any drug.

61. What is immunotherapy and what are its side effects?

Immunotherapy depends on the use of the immune system to treat cancer. Cancer cells may be detected by the immune system; however, they classically cannot as the cancer itself has ways to protect itself from such imminent destruction. Immunotherapy can enhance certain existing antitumor responses or block the protective mechanisms cancer cells may have. Immunotherapy has already been approved for several cancers, including primary liver cancer where nivolumab (Opdivo) received conditional approval and we are awaiting for more data. Nivolumab can be given as a second-line therapy for patients who received prior therapy like sorafenib or lenvatinib. Several other immunotherapies are being evaluated for single agent drug use or in combination with other immunotherapies or biologic and targeted therapies. Immunotherapy like nivolumab can cause shrinkage response in primary liver cancer.

Immunotherapy can be very well tolerated without any side effects; however, relatively uncommon side effects may happen and they can sometimes be serious. Most side effects relate to the overactivation of the immune system; in addition to attacking cancer cells, it can attack other normal organs in the body. Side effects may include fatigue and weakness, rash with possible itching, diarrhea, cough and shortness of breath, and muscle and joint pains. You may develop thyroid deficiency, diabetes, irregular heartbeat, eye inflammation, among other side effects. It is recommended that you report to your doctor any new symptoms as they may be potential side effects to immunotherapy.

62. How will I know that the biologic and targeted therapy or immunotherapy is working? What kind of scan do I need to assess response?

You will take the biologic and targeted therapy or immunotherapy for as long as your doctor finds it helpful in fighting your primary liver cancer. He or she might ask you to stop taking it in case you are not able to tolerate it well. Your doctor will rely on different variables to decide if you are benefiting from taking it. These are mainly your clinical conditions; if you have symptoms, did your symptoms worsen or improve, did new symptoms develop, and the like. In addition, your CT scan or MRI results and AFP level will be considered. All those variables complement each other and your doctor must interpret them to decide if the therapy you are prescribed is benefiting you.

Doctors routinely will use a CT scan, an MRI, or an ultrasound as a baseline before starting any treatment. Because many patients who receive chemotherapy have metastatic disease (stage IV), a CT scan or an MRI of the whole body would be the most reasonable modality to use. You can expect to have a repeat evaluation, preferably using the same radiologic technique, every 2 to 4 months. Any CT scan studying the liver itself should be done using a technique called **triphasic CT** or **four-phase CT scan**. Primary liver cancer lesions are notorious for being difficult to see on a CT scan; however, taking pictures during different phases of the blood flowing through the liver helps the radiologist better interpret the images and any treatment effects.

Triphasic CT
A CT scan that evaluates the liver at three phases of the blood flowing through it.

The radiologic evaluations generally are descriptive. The radiologist can evaluate the cancer in the liver and elsewhere and generally measure it in two dimensions and possibly three. Those measurements are compared with a baseline CT scan or an MRI before the start of therapy and with scans obtained later while on therapy.

Four-phase CT scan
A CT scan that evaluates the liver in four phases as the blood flows through it.

Classically, one might consider that the best result would be a complete response to therapy, where the cancer would disappear completely on the radiologic studies performed. This is extremely unlikely to happen with the treatments discussed for primary liver cancer. However a partial response or reduction in the size of the tumor is likely with lenvatinib and nivolumab. Stable disease may be the best-achieved response with all therapies. Stable disease is a satisfactory response and can justify and support continuing the same treatment. Traditionally and for technical reasons, the category of stable disease is given a margin of 30 percent shrinkage and 20 percent increase in size to accommodate for the technical limitations and other factors of using radiologic tests. Stable disease as a best response to therapy has to do with the way the drug functions, as it is most likely to stabilize the cancer and control it, but not cause it to shrink.

More novel approaches can help assess tumor death, also known as tumor necrosis, and may help identify that the drug is working. Sorafenib was the first to show to cause tumor necrosis; however, the most impressive results have been reported using lenvatinib. Possible necrosis should nonetheless be described as part of your triphasic CT scan report, and your doctor may even quantify it. Obviously, an increase in tumor size of more than 20 percent or the appearance of new tumors represents progression of the disease. This may be a reason to stop the current treatment and to consider a different therapy.

As the immune system can recruit immune cells next to the tumor, tumors may appear to grow rather than shrink, but may ultimately shrink on further follow-up. Thus, your doctor may elect, despite this growth, to keep you on the same drug like nivolumab in view of this pseudoprogression.

63. What about if my liver does not function as well?

There is a serious concern that patients with very advanced cirrhosis (see Questions 22 and 26) may not tolerate any of those biologic and targeted therapies as well as other patients and their cirrhosis may worsen. It is unclear though if this is a direct effect of the drug or simply a worsening of the cirrhosis, which may happen at a faster rate in more severe cases of cirrhosis. Doctors should exert caution in prescribing sorafenib to patients with moderately advanced cirrhosis. They may decide to prescribe it at a lower than recommended starting dose while closely monitoring your liver condition or avoid prescribing it entirely in extremely advanced cases.

64. What is a clinical trial?

A clinical trial is a research study that answers many of the questions regarding newly discovered therapies. Medical researchers discover new therapies daily and describe their mode of action with evolving precision. Over decades, newly discovered therapies must be tested in patients to establish their safety and efficacy.

Clinical trials can answer many scientific and medical questions, which range from testing new drugs, testing a combination of known drugs, and the method of administering certain drugs or testing new therapies such as radiation, nutrition, and behavior. The basic rules, which are discussed later, generally apply to all clinical trials; however, here they are discussed in the context of hepatocellular carcinoma.

A clinical trial is a research study that answers many of the questions regarding newly discovered therapies.

All clinical trials are, and always should be, detailed and clearly described in a manuscript called a protocol. A protocol is the ultimate reference for clinical trials. It describes all of the rules and conditions that govern the trial. This ensures the quality of the trial and thus its reproducibility, as well as the safety and protection of the patients on the trial.

Protocol

A detailed description of all of the rules and conditions that govern a clinical trial. A protocol is the ultimate reference for a clinical trial.

Unfortunately, history tells us about badly conducted clinical trials that might have exploited patients for the sake of answering a scientific question. However, today, patients should not fear joining a clinical trial when clinically indicated, because all **protocols** now are governed by federal regulations that protect all patients. These rules, and many other ethical considerations, are monitored very closely by an **institutional review board**. Patients who are given the option to join a clinical trial make the ultimate decision about whether to participate. If the patient does enter a trial, he or she has the right to withdraw from the trial at any time. These

Institutional review board

A collective board that oversees all clinical trials. The board generally includes doctors, researchers, lawyers, administrators, pharmacists, and patients' advocates.

rights, as well as the details of the study, should be discussed between the patient and the physician in a process called the informed consent, which culminates in both signing an agreement that includes all of the details discussed. This ensures the coherence of the study and protects the rights of all patients.

Clinical trials generally happen in three phases: phase I, II, and III. The goal of a phase I study is primarily to establish the safety of a newly discovered drug or combination of drugs while studying the efficacy in many diseases. A phase II trial studies primarily the efficacy of a drug or a combination of drugs in a specific disease. However, the ultimate answer on efficacy usually is sought through a phase III study, which compares the experimental drug or drugs to the standard care of this disease, such as sorafenib in liver cancer. In a phase III trial, patients will be randomly assigned to either arms of the study (experimental versus standard) to ensure the validity of the experiment. Primary liver cancer is not common in the United States, even though it is one of the most common cancers in the world. A concern exists that its incidence in the United States is on the rise, especially with the increasing prevalence of hepatitis C. This fact and the global aspect of this disease may help bring more awareness and more interest in developing clinical trials.

Not all patients are candidates for clinical trials. Clinical trials are designed to answer specific questions within the boundaries of specific criteria that a certain patient might or might not have. This does not imply that patients who are not eligible for a clinical trial should not be treated.

During the last year of my father's treatment, we explored further options with the doctors, including new chemotherapy drug trials. Unfortunately, by this point, his deteriorating liver health (multiple tumors, ascites, and high blood-protein levels) precluded him from qualifying for many of the trials. Still, that did not prevent me from doing research on the Internet to learn what new phase II and III trials were being offered and whether my father could enroll. I would fax short descriptions of the drug trials to my father's nurse at the clinic and ask her to follow up with doctors before his next scheduled visit. This kept me actively involved in my father's care and offered us hope.

65. Where can I learn about clinical trials for liver cancer, and how do I know which trial is best for me?

Patients should ask their doctors about clinical trials. Many doctors, both at academic centers and in private offices in the community, run or are part of a group of doctors running a clinical trial. Thus, the answer might be at the doorsteps of where a patient lives. Nonetheless, patients might consider commuting a reasonable distance to get to a center that runs a pertinent clinical trial. Patients might know about those through either their doctors, the center's website, or the National Cancer Institute websites: www.cancer.gov and www.clinicaltrials.gov. The National Cancer Institute offers not only a listing of all clinical trials that are registered with them, but also several web pages with information about clinical trials. Other sites that offer similar services include the Coalition of National Cancer Cooperative Groups, www.cancertrialshelp.org, and CenterWatch, www.centerwatch.com.

If a patient identifies a clinical trial that is relevant to his or her medical condition, he or she should discuss the trial further with his or her doctor. The doctor might call the investigators and discover more about the trial. This can ensure that patients will seek only trials that they might be eligible for and save a lot of frustration and travel time and expenses. If a patient is deemed ineligible for a certain trial, he or she should not be disappointed or have feelings of hopelessness. It is important that certain clinical trials answer only a specific question in a specific subset of patients with a given disease. For example, a new drug for primary liver cancer may be tested in only patients who have a specific level of liver function.

It is important to note that this list of clinical trials is very dynamic and could change by the time this book is in print. It is always recommended that you refer to www.clinicaltrials.gov for any updated information about ongoing clinical trials.

66. *Are there any specific new drugs or treatment approaches being tested for primary liver cancer?*

In addition to than the combination approach described in question 61, other novel approaches are underway, especially CAR-T cell therapy. CAR-T cells is short for chimeric antigen receptors (CAR) T cells, which are a patient's T cells that are engineered to target a specific protein on cancer cells. There is quite a bit of interest and excitement for using CAR-T therapy for primary liver cancer and you may be offered such a clinical trial.

67. *What is chemotherapy?*

Cytotoxic drugs

Chemical substances that are used as chemotherapy to kill cancer cells.

Chemotherapy is the use of particular chemicals to kill or arrest the growth of cancer cells. Another name that implies the same function is **cytotoxic drugs** (*cyto* derives from cytology, which is the study of cells). Chemotherapy agents are commonly given intravenously through a needle in the arm, although a few can be given orally as pills. Chemotherapy will thus circulate throughout the body or systemically and not only at selective sites such as the liver. This carries the advantage of treating the cancer at multiple sites in case it has already spread to different sites in the liver or even to the outside of the liver.

Chemotherapy is a generic term that represents a collection of different drugs, just as the word *antibiotics* encompasses a variety of agents that fight bacteria. Not all chemotherapy drugs are the same. Varying drugs are used for varying cancers, and they have different potential side effects. It is important to note that this is a continuously evolving science. Difficult experiences of patients you have heard about from those treated in the past may no longer be the norm, as new chemotherapies with fewer side effects and better supportive medications have been developed.

Chemotherapy is the use of particular chemicals to kill or arrest the growth of cancer cells.

How often chemotherapy is given depends on the drug or combination of drugs based on the nature of the disease and the patient's condition. This does not mean that more frequent delivery of drugs is more effective. A drug may be given in a variety of ways.

Most, if not all, chemotherapy now is given in the outpatient setting. It is rare that you need to be admitted to the hospital to receive chemotherapy. On the day of treatment, you might or might not need to see your medical oncology doctor—depending on where you are in your treatment and how well you are doing. You will have your blood work checked first. This is critically important, because many of the chemotherapy drugs affect your white and red blood cells and platelets (see Question 68). If your blood work shows those cell levels to be in the safe range, then you will proceed to chemotherapy. You will sit in a comfortable chair (such as a recliner), and an IV will be attached to your arm or mediport, if you have one (see Question 81). You will be given a series of some medications, mainly to prevent acute side effects such as nausea, vomiting, diarrhea, or allergic reactions, depending on which drug you are receiving and your previous experience with the drug. Then chemotherapy will be administered. This might take a few minutes to a few hours, depending on which drug is being infused. Some of them may need to be given slowly.

The experience is comfortable. There should be no pain involved. However, if you feel any burning in your arm, you need to tell the nurse immediately, because the IV might have leaked some of the chemotherapy under the skin. You can watch TV, read a magazine—or even read this book—and then have breakfast or lunch after any nausea is under control. At the completion of the chemotherapy, you may need further fluid hydration. At the end of the session, you are disconnected and can go home. You should not drive yourself, because you most likely received some antinausea medicines that could cause drowsiness. Check with your doctor.

68. What are some of the general side effects of chemotherapy?

General side effects can be expected with any chemotherapy treatment, but others are specific to a certain drug or combination of drugs. Because chemotherapy kills reproducing cancer cells, it can be expected that it can kill normal reproducing cells. However, because these normal cells are genetically healthy, they can reproduce again.

Just as chemotherapy might kill dividing cancer cells, it also might harm normal cells in the body that divide rapidly, such as hair follicles, the lining of the guts, and different blood cells. This produces unwanted effects, or toxicity. However, toxicity is reversible, as normal cells have an inherent ability to repair and replace the destroyed cells—something cancer cells commonly cannot do because they lack repair mechanisms.

An expected general side effect of chemotherapy is the destruction of **red blood cells** that carry oxygen, **white blood cells** that fight infections, and **platelets** that are responsible for clotting blood. The caring physician should be monitoring these carefully through routine blood work. Patients will be cautioned at the same time to mention extra signs of fatigue. Though fatigue may be explained by a lower number of red blood cells, not all fatigue symptoms are due to this. Patients with primary liver cancer might be tired because of their illness, and the chemotherapy itself undoubtedly might cause tiredness. Infections are possible because of reduced white cells. Any sign of fever should prompt a call to the physician and even a possible visit to the hospital. A physician again might elect to give a certain skin injection to boost the number of white cells. This is not necessarily done even if the white count is low, because it depends on the chemotherapy scheduling and some other factors. Bleeding through the mouth, rectum, or other sites is of critical importance, especially in primary liver cancer, where the number of platelets could be low to start with because of liver failure or cirrhosis. Physicians might elect to give chemotherapy for patients with platelet levels that are lower than the commonly used reference of 100,000 per mcL; however, this requires extreme vigilance by both the patient and physician.

Red blood cells

Cells that carry oxygen and carbon dioxide. They are red because of their high load of iron, which is essential to their function.

White blood cells

Cells that help fight infection.

Platelets

Pieces of cells that float in the blood and promote clotting where necessary.

Several chemotherapy agents cause nausea and possibly vomiting, but to variable extents. Because these symptoms are predictable, patients most likely will be taught about the potential nausea and will be given supportive medications to prevent or alleviate it. Several new, very effective antinausea medicines are now readily available. One form of nausea is anticipatory that a patient might have learned due to poor control of nausea and/or vomiting with previous chemotherapy treatments. This stresses the importance of controlling nausea as tightly as possible. The good thing is that there are now many drugs to help with even severe nausea. Other side effects include abdominal pain and tingling sensation or sometimes pain in the fingers and toes. Most importantly, it is very difficult to know or tell how you may react to chemotherapy. Patients may have none of those side effects, all of them, or some of them. In anticipation, it is good to learn about all that might happen and inform your doctor of any symptoms that seem unusual or unexpected.

As the drug is being infused, patients should notify the nurses immediately if they experience any pain, discoloration, or burning at the infusion site.

69. Which chemotherapy drugs might be used to treat liver cancer?

The National Comprehensive Cancer Center Network does not list any chemotherapy agent as a standard of care for primary liver cancer. Doxorubicin (Adriamycin) was the first and remains the most studied chemotherapy in primary liver cancer. Doxorubicin was never established as a standard of care for this disease and thus should not be used.

A more novel therapy called FOLFOX proved to be more valuable and effective than doxorubicin. FOLFOX consists of three drugs, 5-flurouracil (Adrucil), oxaliplatin (Eloxatin), and leucovorin. You would receive the oxaliplatin and leucovorin as infusions in the clinic along with a starter bolus of 5-flurouracil. You will then be connected through the mediport (see Question 81) to a bag that has 2 days worth of 5-flurouracil that you will have infused at home. You will then return to the clinic to be disconnected from the bag. In time you may be taught to disconnect yourself at home.

FOLFOX is already an approved standard of care of therapy for primary liver cancer in China. While it is not approved in other places, your doctor may elect to treat you with this regimen as the drugs are already available to treat other cancers.

70. Is receiving more than one chemotherapy drug better?

Many attempts have been made to improve on the efficacy of single-agent doxorubicin by adding other drugs. Other drug combinations without doxorubicin also have been tested. The only combination that has been tested in a phase III trial against single-agent doxorubicin is doxorubicin plus cisplatin (Platinol), 5-fluorouracil, and interferon—a combination that is known as PIAF. Overall, results do not support the routine use of PIAF. This is especially true in view of the extensive toxicity that might develop from using this combination of therapy including possible hospitalization because of reduced immunity, reduction in white blood cells, and fever, which may require treatment with antibiotics and other supportive medications. However, a careful interpretation of these data and data from a phase II study of the same combination justifies using PIAF in some patients who might benefit from chemotherapy in an aim to shrink their tumor and render it resectable by surgery, a process called neoadjuvant therapy. Such a strategy should be considered carefully where applicable, and any decision should involve a medical oncologist and a surgeon. Another approach involving adding drugs to FOLFOX is underway.

71. What is liver pump chemotherapy?

Some patients might have cancer in only the liver that is, however, scattered throughout the liver. This situation, as explained earlier, would not be amenable to surgery, transplant, or any other of the local therapies previously discussed. However, the chemotherapy might be given only where needed in the liver, thus maximizing its effectiveness against the disease and minimizing any possible systemic side effects. This therapy entails having a simple catheter inserted into an artery that leads to your liver, through which chemotherapy is given. Another possibility is having a **pump** placed under the skin in the wall of your abdomen; it is connected in the same way to an artery that leads to the liver. The pump can be accessed through the skin like the mediport (see Question 81). The drug that is administered through the pump will be delivered to your liver, but it will be over a longer period of time—generally 2 weeks—thus exposing the tumor to more chemotherapy.

Pump

A pump system used to deliver chemotherapy at a fixed rate and for a specific period of time.

Many studies have been done about this form of therapy; however, until now, at least in the United States, this is not considered a standard of care. The results have not been that promising to date so this treatment should only be used as part of a clinical trial.

72. What is radiation therapy?

Radiation therapy

Treatment against cancer that uses radiation as a form of energy to kill cancer cells.

Radiation therapy depends on the high energy of certain electromagnetic waves. These powerful radiation rays can be controlled and directed toward a cancer. The aim is obviously to kill cancer cells. The two main types of radiation waves are x-rays and gamma-rays. They differ in production and power, and may have different applicability in cancer treatment. Radiation can be delivered from outside of the body, penetrate through the skin, and be targeted to where the tumor is. This is called **external beam radiation**; it usually consists of x-rays. Another form of radiation that produces gamma-rays from radioactive material can be inserted or implanted inside the body next to where the tumor is. This is called **brachytherapy**.

External beam radiation

Radiation therapy that is aimed at a specific site in the body and delivered from outside of the body through the skin.

Brachytherapy

Radiation therapy that is applied within the body cavity.

73. Can radiation be used to treat liver cancer?

Although radiation is a commonly used form of treatment for many cancers, its role in the case of primary liver cancer is rather limited because the liver has poor tolerance to radiation. Generally, the number of treatments to the liver will not be more than 10. These usually are delivered daily Monday to Friday over 1 week. Radiating the entire liver might cause liver inflammation, called **radiation hepatitis**. Today, this problem can be overcome by using localized radiation therapy to where it is needed in the liver. Doctors who treat cancer patients with radiation (also called radiation oncologists) can prepare a three-dimensional computer model of the liver and the tumor. They then target a small radiation therapy emitted from many sources to a very localized focus of the tumor where the effect of the sum of all those small amounts of radiation will maximize and cause tumor damage without affecting the surrounding liver tissue. Because of the limitations of radiation in liver cancer, the role of radiation therapy in hepatocellular carcinoma is limited to palliation and control of pain, if any. Another use of radiation in primary liver cancer is to help relieve pain at sites where the cancer has spread to the bone. It also may be used preventively

Radiation hepatitis

Inflammatory damage to the liver that may be caused by radiation therapy.

to avoid a bone fracture at a weak site where the cancer has spread (e.g., hips). One other use of radiation is to reduce the size of cancer sites in the vertebral bodies to prevent them from compressing the spinal cord and causing nerve paralysis. This is an emergency condition that should be avoided at every cost because the patient may become paralyzed if this is to occur. If at any time you develop any arm or leg weakness, especially if it is one sided; have a decreased sensation in any of the extremities; or if you lose urine or stools uncontrollably or without knowing, you need to call your doctor immediately because these may be signs of a spinal cord compression by cancer that requires immediate attention. Treatments include the possibility of either surgery or radiation, plus steroids that are given to help reduce any inflammation that may contribute to the symptoms.

Although radiation is a commonly used form of treatment for many cancers, its role in the case of primary liver cancer is rather limited because the liver has poor tolerance to radiation.

74. What are yttrium-90 microspheres?

New advances in radiation have expanded its use in hepatocellular carcinoma. Today, highly potent radioactive material can be attached to glass beads that can be infused into the hepatic artery and lodge next to and into the tumors that are regularly fed by the hepatic artery.

Yttrium-90 microspheres, also known as Therasphere, have been studied in the liver since the late 1980s and have been proven to be active in multiple clinical trials. Several trials compared yttrium-90 microspheres to sorafenib for advanced HCC, and others looked into the combination of yttrium-90 microspheres plus sorafenib, but none have shown a survival advantage over sorafenib. Thus yttrium-90 microspheres may be recommended as a local therapy for locally advanced disease but not for advanced disease with metastasis (spread out disease). A variety of smaller studies are

Yttrium-90 microspheres

Small beads tagged with radioactive yttrium that are delivered into the liver and lodge inside the small arteries to deliver their anticancer therapeutic effect.

examining sterotactic radiation plus sorafenib and proton beam radiation plus sorafenib. Again, all those approaches are still investigational and should not be used outside of clinical trial settings until safety and efficacy data are reported. You can visit www.clinicaltrials.gov to learn more about those studies.

75. What are the side effects of radiation?

The side effects of radiation therapy depend on the part of the body that is being irradiated. After radiating the liver, the overlying skin will be the first to be damaged by the radiation. You may notice it to be darker and dry, both over the abdomen and the back. Rarely, the skin might burn and appear red. The liver itself, as mentioned already, may sustain further damage secondary to radiation. This will be critical, especially if it is already cirrhotic. The closeness to the stomach might cause nausea, vomiting, and irritation of the lining of the stomach. You also may get diarrhea, because the radiation might affect the lining of the bowels, which are in close proximity to the field of radiation. Radiation generally causes tiredness and fatigue. Finally, patients might have reduced white cells, red cells, or platelets because the radiation might injure their production site in the bone marrow in the vertebral column lying right behind the liver.

Complementary medicine

A method of health care that combines the therapies and philosophies of conventional medicine with those of alternative medicines.

Alternative medicine

Healthcare and treatment practices, including traditional Chinese medicine, chiropractic, folk medicine, and naturopathy, that minimize or eschew the use of surgery and drugs.

76. What are complementary and alternative treatments?

Complementary medicine and **alternative medicine** are acknowledged by the National Institutes of Health and the health system as another approach to therapy that would help integrate such unconventional treatments with more conventional therapies. Many cancer centers around the country now have an integrative medicine department or a section that offers alternative therapies to patients. These include, but are not limited to, alternative systems of medical practice such as **acupuncture**, **homeopathy**, and **naturopathy**. Diet and nutrition are other components. For the mind and body, many places offer psychotherapy, meditation, hypnosis, biofeedback, and massage, among many others. You also may seek herbal remedies and other medicines that are still considered alternative by nature because they lack a clear indication by Western medicine standards.

Acupuncture

A Chinese medical procedure in which fine needles are placed through the skin to relieve pain or for other treatment reasons.

Homeopathy

Treating disease with small amounts of treatments that in large amounts in healthy people may produce symptoms of the same disease.

Naturopathy

The science that uses herbs and herb products as a form of therapy against disease.

A great deal of research has undoubtedly proven some of these therapies to be effective. Discuss your interest in these methods with your doctor, who might refer you to an integrative medicine doctor. Avoid taking any medicines on your own unless you discuss it with your doctor. Remember that many of today's medicines are of natural origins. By the same token, many of the medicines that are labeled as natural or herbal can have potential effects and even side effects. More importantly, your doctor might help you to identify the therapies that you should avoid. Oncologists know more about alternative therapies than before and may expect their patients to use them. Do not hesitate to discuss alternative therapies with your doctors. Bring the pills and herbs with you, and always try to have a list of ingredients. This might help your doctor to identify any potentially beneficial or harmful products.

After 3 years of relatively stable health, my father's condition took a precipitous dive and he had to be rushed to the hospital because of infection and sludge buildup in his gallbladder. It was around then that his CT scans showed tumor growth in one of his adrenal glands. The chemotherapy regimen did not seem to be working. At that point, my family and I started to seek alternative treatments because his conventional options seemed to be running out.

Many websites and family friends touted the antitumor properties of mushrooms such as Agaricus blazei Murrill, *and Maitake. Although the anecdotal evidence was very encouraging, the clinical studies, mostly in Japanese and Chinese journals, supporting these treatments are very limited at best. The theories propose that the mushrooms contain certain polysaccharides that strengthen the immune system's fight against cancer. I would advise everyone to be careful about the optimistic claims, because most are being promoted by the supplement manufacturers themselves.*

After consulting with his doctors, we did give my father various mushroom extracts, along with milk thistle, an herb that is supposed to improve liver function. We figured their potential negative side effects were small. We also tried a very risky liquid cesium treatment but stopped it after 2 weeks when my father's digestive system did not tolerate it very well. It is unknown whether these alternative treatments were beneficial to his health.

Complementary medicine and alternative medicine are acknowledged by the National Institutes of Health and the health system as another approach to therapy that would help integrate such unconventional treatments with more conventional therapies.

77. What if my doctor recommends that no treatment should be performed?

Some patients are not eligible for any of the previously discussed treatments. Your doctor may decide that it is too risky to treat you if your tumor is too advanced, if your liver is too weak because of advanced stage cirrhosis, or if you have other significant medical problems. In this situation, your doctor will offer the best supportive care. You should not perceive this approach as if your doctor or you are giving up. This approach might provide protection against things that might get worse, like the cirrhosis, should you be treated. This means that he or she will try to help with any symptoms that you may develop and try to maximize your quality of life. In particular, he or she will help you try to prevent further liver failure or complications from cirrhosis. This is done by helping you to avoid gaining extra fluid weight by using diuretics (water pills). Other symptoms that may require treatment include mental confusion and bleeding from your stomach. You may not necessarily experience any pain, but if you do, pain medications can and should be prescribed. Some patients also may require assistance with living at home, and often a social worker can help arrange for a healthcare professional to visit you.

I believe that doctors correctly wanted to avoid doing harm to my father; thus, they stopped his treatments when they did not look like they were working. The liver is a complex chemical factory, and during cancer treatment, it is in a precarious balance. My family and I eventually came to realize that our doctors were more focused on sustaining his quality of life rather than grasping at dangerous straws for a cure.

78. How should I use the Internet to learn about my cancer?

The Internet has a vast resource of medical information. You may learn about a specialty center near you or discover a clinical trial in which you can participate. Although many doctors recommend that you learn about your cancer, they will caution you that many times a patient will find information that is not relevant to their particular situation. This may lead to further confusion or fear. Thus, although it is valuable for you and your family to learn about HCC, you should discuss your Internet research with your doctor. The value of a certain website will depend on some aspects, including the accuracy of the information. Remember that some sites

Although it is valuable for you and your family to learn about HCC, you should discuss your Internet research with your doctor.

are more reputable than others. Look at who is behind the website and learn whether there is supporting staff you can contact for any questions. Make sure though that your confidentiality as a patient is kept while navigating any such sources on the Internet. The Internet also may enable you to communicate with other patients who have your disease, which may help you cope with the problems that you are facing. However, you must be cautious about certain chat rooms, because many are not monitored, and any data or information you might gather needs to be placed in context.

PART SEVEN

Cancer-Related Practical Issues

I feel overwhelmed by all of the information that I am receiving. How do I make any decisions regarding my treatment?

Will changing my diet alter my cancer?

What is a mediport?

More . . .

79. I feel overwhelmed by all of the information that I am receiving. How do I make any decisions regarding my treatment?

This sentiment is understandable and expected after you have read the previous sections of this book and realized that there are many different approaches to therapy. That's good in a way, to know that there are many resources available to help. The best way to incorporate this information is to keep track of it. Take notes, but do not immerse yourself in details because you might lose the big picture this way. In many cancer centers, you might be followed by many physicians. Your doctors will be talking to each other. It is a good idea, however, to identify one physician as the primary caring one, for example, your surgeon in case your prime therapy is a surgery or your medical oncologist if you are receiving systemic therapy. The addition of sorafenib to the different therapies now available for patients with primary liver cancer, and the expected increase in new information available about other therapies and combination of different therapies may overwhelm you as well. The best advice that remains is to ask your doctor to clarify matters but always keep it in the context of your personal medical situation. Reported details from specific clinical studies should always be interpreted in the context of that big picture.

I felt that one of the most exasperating experiences of my father's cancer was figuring out who was in charge. Because liver cancer currently has no single default method of care, but instead many avenues of treatment, during each trip to the clinic, we would have to talk to the surgeon about surgery options, the radiologist about the embolization treatment options, the oncologist about chemotherapy options, the hepatobiliary specialist about hepatitis options, and so forth, and then we would try to assimilate all of the information ourselves. In retrospect, we maybe should have tried harder to identify a primary physician early on for my father—someone among the specialists involved who is fairly well-versed in the disease and could coordinate care among all of the other specialists.

80. Will changing my diet alter my cancer?

This is a common question among patients with cancer. In general, no specific diet recommendations are available for cancer patients and most doctors would encourage you to eat a balanced diet. While proteins are always encouraged to regain muscle mass, in the specific setting of liver cancer, your doctor might caution you and your family that eating too much protein might make you sleepy or confused, and thus a certain amount may be needed to help you add weight but avoid mental status changes (see Question 92). Your doctor may advise taking one multivitamin pill a day but most likely will advise against an intense vitamin and herbal therapy, especially if your liver already is jeopardized by the cancer and possible cirrhosis. You should try to eliminate alcohol use. If you have cirrhosis, your doctor may limit the amount of fluid that you drink or the salt and protein that you eat. Your doctor may recommend that you seek advice from a hepatologist or a nutritionist.

As my father's cancer progressed, it became more and more difficult for him to do simple things such as swallowing foods and pills. His sense of taste also was changing. Nearly all foods lacked flavor, and he would crave a lot of salt or spice, which we tried to avoid.

In response, we would try to prepare a few foods that he liked as a special treat, such as pizza, while still encouraging him to eat the bland, healthy foods that he did not like, such as vegetables and beans. Because he had difficulty swallowing pills, we found liquid multivitamins (available online) to supplement his diet.

You may wonder about the consumption of sugar in the setting of the cancer. This is yet to be confirmed and validated. Your doctor is less likely to recommend such dietary limitation.

81. What is a mediport?

Mediport

A half-dollar sized, round well that is connected to a tube that is used for the delivery of medication within a vein. The entire apparatus sits underneath the skin and is inserted during a small procedure.

A **mediport** is a device that can be used to deliver chemotherapy. It may be necessary if the patient has limited intravenous access in the arms or if the chemotherapy is to be delivered continuously while the patient is at home. A mediport is inserted underneath the skin of your chest wall by a surgeon or an interventional radiologist. The procedure takes about 45 minutes and is performed while you are lightly sedated.

A mediport has two components: a reservoir and a tube. Both are underneath your skin. The reservoir is about the width of a half dollar. It may be visible as a small lump just below your collarbone. A nurse inserts a needle through your skin into the reservoir. The drug, or any other intravenous solution, then passes into a small tube that sits inside a large vein in your body.

Three main complications of having a mediport exist. The first is that during the insertion of the device, there is an approximate 1 percent chance of having one of your lungs collapse. This is treated by placing a small tube into the chest and removing some air. The more common complications include infection and a blood clot. Because a mediport is a foreign object in your body, it might become infected. Thus, it is critical that there is an indication for a mediport and that it is not just inserted for convenience. Also, only an experienced person should access the mediport, and it should be done in a sterile fashion. Because the catheter attached to the reservoir sits in a vein, this vein may develop a clot. Your doctor may request that you take a very small dose of a blood thinner called warfarin (Coumadin) while you have a mediport. If either an infection or a blood clot occurs, your mediport may need to be removed.

82. Why are my eyes and/or skin yellow?

Jaundice is caused by the accumulation of bile in the body (see Question 22). It is a complication of liver failure and cirrhosis. The liver cells may be destroyed and release an overwhelming amount of bile that your body cannot absorb like it normally does, thus causing you to look yellow. By itself, jaundice is not dangerous, and at worst, it may cause itching that can be treated with a medicine such as Benadryl. However, the presence of jaundice is a sign of a failing liver, and it could prevent you from having a surgery or receiving therapy, because this may further worsen your liver condition. Jaundice also might occur or worsen while receiving therapy (e.g., sorafenib; see Question 61) especially if you have an advanced stage of cirrhosis and you receive the drug. It is unclear though if this is due to the drug itself or part of the natural progression of the cirrhosis. Clearly, additional data is needed in this regard. Until then, your doctor might elect to not give you sorafenib with the fear of a worsening in your condition rather than an improvement. Another cause of jaundice is a mechanical block in the liver that is caused by the tumor. The tumor may press on a bile duct and not allow the bile to drain the normal way into your gallbladder and intestine; thus, it backs up in the liver and causes jaundice. In this case, your doctors may recommend a diverting procedure for the bile in order to decrease it and be able to treat you with chemotherapy or to relieve you of any symptoms such as severe itching.

83. How can a mechanical blockage of bile be fixed?

Gastroenterologist

A doctor who specializes in the treatment of diseases that affect the gastrointestinal system, including the liver, stomach, and pancreas.

There are several ways to fix a blocked bile duct. One is to have a plastic or metal stent placed into your bile duct during an endoscopy. A **gastroenterologist** performs an endoscopy while you are lightly sedated. A scope is put through your mouth into your intestine. The stent is fed through the bile duct opening in your intestine. The other main way to fix a bile duct blockage is by placing a plastic tube (called a catheter) directly through your abdominal wall into the liver and then through the bile duct. Initially, bile will drain into a bag that you may place at a lower point of its insertion site under your clothes, around your waist, or around your leg. The procedure is performed by a team of interventional radiologists while you are lightly sedated. For this, you may be admitted to the hospital and observed for a few days. It may take several days for your bilirubin level to drop low enough for you to start chemotherapy again. One of the risks of the procedure is infection; thus, you may need to be treated with antibiotics intravenously. Other complications include bleeding. This is of special concern in patients with advanced cirrhosis, because their blood may not clot normally. This by itself may even prevent you from having the procedure. In many instances, the interventional radiologist may soon be able to place the stent permanently on the inside so that you do not have to have a bag.

84. I feel tired. Can I do anything about it?

Fatigue is a common symptom for patients with cancer. This is due to many factors. The cancer itself, especially in its advanced stages, might tire people. In addition, systemic therapy (e.g., sorafenib) might cause fatigue, which may require an adjustment of the dose of the drug you are given. Some chemotherapy might cause a drop in the number of your red blood cells, which also can contribute to fatigue. Your doctor may recommend, in uncommon instances, an injection that stimulates your body to produce more red blood cells (e.g., epoetin alfa [Procrit] or darbepoetin alfa [Aranesp]). This might not relieve all of the fatigue but might make you feel better. In addition, despite its value, your doctor most likely will advise against it or give it only when you have specifically very low levels of red blood cells. This is important because new data has come out about the negative impact of red blood stimulation agents, including but not limited to, increased death, serious heart problems, and cancer progression.

The liver cells may be destroyed and release an overwhelming amount of bile that your body cannot absorb like it normally does, thus causing you to look yellow.

Mental fatigue is another symptom. It results from all of the doctor appointments, tests, and the concerns and fears of having cancer. Mental fatigue is best circumvented by focusing on the daily goals and keeping notes of events so that you do not burden yourself with all of the information that you are getting. Keep it simple, and remember to always look at the big picture. Many relatives, friends, and colleagues will be calling to check on you. It is very good to have people around, and your doctors will always encourage you to maintain your social support group. It is okay not to think about your cancer all of the time. You need to energize and be ready for the next step all the time.

Pain is another cause of fatigue. You have to make sure it is well controlled, as is discussed in Question 85.

Fatigue is a common symptom for patients with cancer.

I discovered simple activities that helped to revive my dad's energy and spirits. We would take short walks around the house, making it a game of how many times he could circle the kitchen before getting too tired. We rented DVDs of his favorite movies. We played board games and cards. These seemed to help take his mind off his fatigue. Even so, he took naps more frequently and complained of sore, tired muscles, particularly the upper arms, shoulders, and legs.

85. I have pain. How can I be pain free?

Nonsteroidal anti-inflammatory drugs

A form of medication that controls pain and inflammation that is not part of the steroid family.

Pain needs to be controlled, because it might affect your mood and your function and cause you to be more ill, tired, and fatigued. You have to tell your doctor about pain because it can be alleviated. Mild pains usually respond to acetaminophen (Tylenol) or **nonsteroidal anti-inflammatory drugs** (NSAIDs) such as ibuprofen (Motrin and Advil). Acetaminophen should, however, be taken gingerly because it might affect liver function, especially in the case of advanced cirrhosis. Make sure that you tell your doctor how many acetaminophen you need and have him or her assess its safety. The NSAIDs might cause stomach bleeding, which is possible because of the cirrhosis (see Question 89). These medications may not be enough to control your pain.

In case of more severe pain, you may be prescribed opiate- or morphine-based medications. Many formulations of those medications exist; they are divided into two main categories: short-acting and long-acting. If you may require only a few pills daily or every few days to control your pain, your doctor most likely will prescribe a short-acting morphine such as oxycodone, one to two pills every 4 to 6 hours. These will control your pain for that period of time. Some of the short-acting opiates are a combination of Tylenol plus oxycodone (Oxycontin), such as Percocet. Your doctor may avoid prescribing those for the same concerns raised with the Tylenol; that is, liver function. If you require many short-acting pills to control pain, your doctor may elect to add a long-acting opiate that can be in the form of pills like Oxycontin, or morphine (MS Contin) that you take twice a day, or as a skin patch (fentanyl [Actiq]) that you apply every 3 days. Although the patch appears to be easier, you still may be prescribed pills because of allergic concerns, personal preference, or sometimes poor absorption because of reduced body fat.

The aim is to be pain free. You have to bear in mind that your pain medications requirements may increase with time because of a totally natural phenomenon called **tolerance** (this should not be mistaken with addiction); also, your pain may simply get worse, and you need more medications to control it. Some patients with liver cirrhosis and liver cancer who may have acquired hepatitis through shared needles for drug use may feel uncomfortable using opiates. You are strongly encouraged to speak about your fears and concerns, because assistance from your medical oncologist or even pain specialist should be available.

Tolerance

The body's need for an increased dose of a certain medication to obtain the same effect.

Like all medications, opiates have side effects. You may feel sleepy or drowsy, especially at first. This may dissipate after a few days. If it persists, your medications may need to be fine tuned to reach a comfortable pain-control level, with acceptable side effects.

In all instances, however, you should not operate any machinery or drive while taking opiates. In more advanced medical situations, where you might require a high dose of pain medications, you may sleep for long periods of time. While this may be concerning for your family and friends who would like to see you awake and conversing with them, pain control should be favored. Constipation is another side effect. Your bowels may become a bit sluggish while on opiates, and most likely you will need to be maintained on a daily bowel regimen of a stool softener such as Colace) and a laxative such as Senekot, Miralax, magnesium citrate, or Lactulose. Drinking fluids also will help keep you regular. You may have more or fewer side effects with different formulations of opiates. Sometimes switching to different medications may help ease some of the side effects.

Cirrhosis-Related Practical Issues

My legs and/or my abdomen are swollen. What can I do about it?

What is meant when my platelets are low?

I am vomiting or passing blood and coffee-ground material in my stool. What is causing this?

More . . .

86. My legs and/or my abdomen are swollen. What can I do about it?

In the event of cirrhosis, blood pressure might build up inside the liver, causing what is called portal hypertension. This causes the body to start accumulating more water and salt, which ultimately leads to swelling in the abdomen (ascites) or in the legs (peripheral edema). The reduced ability of the cirrhotic liver to produce protein, in addition to poor nutrition, which usually is associated with cirrhosis and/or primary liver cancer, also may contribute to the swelling. When the blood vessels have a reduced amount of protein in them, they cannot retain water as well. Thus, water will seep out of the blood vessels and cause ascites and **edema**.

Edema

An abnormal accumulation of fluid in the extremities.

As you can imagine, resolution of the fluid is unlikely to happen unless the cirrhosis improves, which may not be possible. Still, your doctor might be able to help reduce the amount of accumulating fluid. The simplest way would be to restrict salt intake, because salt draws water with it. You might need to restrict your salt intake to less than 2 grams of salt (800 mg of sodium) per day; as an example, one slice of bread has about 0.5 gram of salt. Your doctor also may prescribe a water pill (diuretic) such as spironolactone (Aldactone) or a combination of diuretics by adding furosemide (Lasix). Usually such interventions would be sufficient to keep the fluid retention at a steady level. However, sometimes your doctor might need to remove the fluid or ascites from your abdomen by inserting a needle through the skin. This is a simple bedside procedure that could be done with or without the help of an ultrasound to localize the fluid. During the procedure, you lie on your back, probably turning more toward your right. Your doctor will sterilize one spot of your skin, usually in the left lower corner of your abdomen. You then will receive numbing medicine through a needle. Afterward, your doctor will insert a needle with a catheter that will drain the clear yellowish fluid into a bottle or a bag. Your doctor will judge how much fluid should be removed to make sure that your blood pressure and other vital signs are not affected by this rapid change of body fluid. The procedure carries a small risk of infection or bleeding (see Question 87) and also might make you lose some of your good proteins.

The management of ascites and edema is a very difficult task. In a situation with more advanced cirrhosis, they may be even impossible to control; pain control may be the only approach that helps to alleviate discomfort.

For my father, a low dosage of spironolactone helped to keep his ascites and edema in check most of the time. During the advanced phase of his cancer, we found that support socks helped to reduce the swelling in his lower legs and feet. They are available in different ranges of compression (we used moderate) at most drug stores. We would help him put them on, rolling them up just past his knees. His only complaint was that they were uncomfortably hot sometimes, especially at night. Massaging the feet and ankles is another good way to help maintain flexibility.

87. What is meant when my platelets are low?

Platelets are small cell parts that help the blood to form a clot. Portal hypertension (see Question 86) might cause blood to back up into the **spleen**, which then starts enlarging to accommodate for the increased blood flow. The spleen typically entraps platelets, and with a larger spleen, more platelets will lodge there. This will lead to a reduced amount of platelets in the blood. A more novel understanding indicates that platelets may be reduced due to

Spleen

An organ located in the upper left part of the abdomen that filters toxic foreign substances from the blood. In case of liver failure, the spleen may enlarge.

the reduction in a hormone that help produce them that is made in the liver. It is unclear why this would happen and if it a good or bad effect of the disease. On one hand, an improvement in the platelets may sound great, however potential clotting can increase. Interestingly some research work has shown that patients with low platelets may fare better on sorafenib (Nexavar) than patients with high platelet levels. In general, not much can be done to improve your platelet count. Certain hormones can be given to improve the platelets number, but this may cause more clotting. You doctor will judge what is most appropriate to do. however, stable and well-controlled cirrhosis and portal hypertension may improve the platelet count somewhat. Alcohol should be completely avoided to prevent the cirrhosis from worsening and further reducing the platelet count.

The low platelet count might limit the kind of diagnostic procedures or therapies that you might be offered because of the increased risk of bleeding. Your doctor might feel that it isn't safe to have a biopsy to diagnose your cancer. This is acceptable because with low platelets you might not be eligible to receive an embolization or systemic therapy (e.g., because of the risk of bleeding). This is especially important in the case of sorafenib or a drug from the same category of drugs that disrupt the blood supply to the tumor (see Question 60), which also may make patients more prone to bleeding. In that instance, caring for your cirrhosis would be of utmost importance.

88. I am vomiting or passing blood and coffee-ground material in my stool. What is causing this?

The high-pressure buildup caused by portal hypertension might lead to the development of collateral blood vessels called varices in many body organs, such as the esophagus and stomach. These collaterals, however, are at a risk of bleeding as the high pressure is also transmitted through them. The esophageal and stomach varices might open up and bleed, causing you to vomit blood or coffee-ground material. You may have bloody or dark stools as well. This is an emergency that requires immediate medical attention. If you witness any of these symptoms, please call your doctor or any emergency medical service immediately. You might feel a rapid heart beat because your heart is trying to compensate for the lost blood, and you might faint. The bleeding might not stop and might require immediate medical intervention.

89. How can I stop the bleeding?

If you happen to have a variceal bleed, time is of the essence. In the emergency room, you will be transfused with blood and plasma to replace the blood that you lost and to help your blood to clot. Depending on the severity of the episode, your gastroenterologist or hepatologist might elect to perform an endoscopy to locate the bleeding varices and inject them or band them in an attempt to stop or prevent recurrence of the bleeding. Other interventions also might be needed.

In all instances, you might already have been, or you will be prescribed different medications to help reduce your risk of bleeding or to stop the bleeding when it happens.

90. I think I am yellow or that my eyes are yellow. What does that mean?

If a mechanical blockage of your bile duct is not present, then jaundice (see Questions 22 and 82) usually is a sign of advanced liver failure or cirrhosis. Liver destruction leads to further accumulation of bile that will show as increased bilirubin and jaundice. As cirrhosis advances, the bilirubin or jaundice worsen (see Question 28). In most cases, not much can be done to reverse this jaundice, except possibly liver transplantation (see Question 47). However, your doctor might prescribe antihistamines such as Atarax or Benadryl to ease any itching that you might have. These medications might make you sleepy though. This sleepiness could become important and should be carefully assessed as not to confuse it with any symptoms that are directly related to cirrhosis (see Question 91).

Coma

Loss of consciousness that may occur when the liver is no longer working well.

91. My family or people surrounding me are stating that I am confused or sleepy sometimes. What is causing this?

The cirrhotic liver might not be able to process many toxic substances, which will accumulate in the blood and may circulate through the brain and alter your mental status.

The cirrhotic liver might not be able to process many toxic substances, which will accumulate in the blood and may circulate through the brain and alter your mental status. You might be confused or sleepy at times; you might have personality changes. In advanced cases, patients may fall into a **coma**. These symptoms are collectively called encephalopathy. They might happen gradually and over a long period of time or more acutely, depending on the evolvement of the liver disease. You and your family should keep your doctor updated regarding any signs or symptoms that relate to disturbed level of awareness, episodes of forgetfulness, confusion, personality changes, seizures, or any other concern you might have because some treatments might help this condition (see Question 92).

92. How can I think more clearly?

To improve the encephalopathy, therapy is aimed to reduce the amount of toxins you might have in your body. **Ammonia** is among the most notorious substances that lead to this condition, but not necessarily the only one. You may be prescribed lactulose (Duphalac), a laxative that will reduce the amount of protein and nitrogen-based substances absorbed through your intestines. The amount of lactulose that you need can be gauged by the number of stools that you have per day. You should aim at two to four soft bowel movements per day. In addition, you might be asked to restrict the amount of protein you take for the same reason. This can pose a delicate issue when it comes to balancing your need for nutrition. Your doctor will help you balance the two by prescribing a preset amount of protein that you can take per day. Your doctor can follow your improvement not only clinically as your symptoms improve, but also by measuring your blood ammonia level. In advanced cancer situations, especially if you happen to be in hospice care, the effect of the ammonia may help sedate you and control your pain. Therefore, treating your sedation may not necessarily be required.

Ammonia

A body of excreted substances that normally is broken down by the liver.

PART NINE

Social and End-of-Life Issues

Can my liver cancer be transmitted to my family?

Can I work while getting treated?

What if my doctors suggest stopping my current therapy?

More . . .

93. Can my liver cancer be transmitted to my family?

Although the hepatitis virus can be transmitted by patients with active disease, scientists have no evidence that HCC can be contagious. Your family members should be reassured that they will not develop cancer by being around you. If you have a genetic disease that caused your cancer (see Box 2), then your children should be screened for the disease. Your doctor should discuss this with you.

94. Can I work while getting treated?

Most patients with primary liver cancer can return to work after surgery, liver transplant, or a local therapy such as embolization. Also, many patients who are receiving chemotherapy can continue going to work. If your body allows and you are not tired, go to work to keep a sense of normalcy in your life. You may be able to work only part time, because you may need a few days after treatment to rest and recover. In all instances, make sure to discuss your interests and concerns with your doctor. If you are working, you are most likely entitled to sick days or even an unpaid leave. You can check the U.S. Department of Labor Medical Leave Act of 1993 at https://www.dol.gov/whd/fmla/. You also may need to review your disability benefits. The benefits department at your place of employment should be able to discuss all of the benefits to which you are entitled.

You may be concerned to tell your supervisor or coworkers about your diagnosis of cancer. It is definitely a personal preference regarding how much information you want to share. However, more importantly, you should not fear being treated differently or being discriminated against. The American with Disabilities Act clearly states your rights and protects you against discrimination at work. It also requires that employers make reasonable adjustments as long as you can perform the essential functions of your job. You may need to discuss your work schedule, limitations, and other aspects of your job with the Human Resource department. In case of a conflict, you may need to contact your lawyer or the U.S. Department of Justice at 800-514-0301 or at www.ada.gov.

Remember that your supervisor and coworkers may feel uncomfortable knowing about your diagnosis, either because of previous family experience or because of fear of a disease that they do not know much about. For those who are interested, try to educate them; for those who decide to alienate you, remain kind and courteous. With time, as they see you functioning like any other person, their fears and anxieties may dissipate, and the relationship may normalize.

95. What if my doctors suggest stopping my current therapy?

If the cancer becomes too advanced and resistant to therapy, or if your body becomes too weak to tolerate any treatment, your doctor may elect to stop all active therapies. You may be angry or upset or feel helpless about that. However, your doctor is definitely not giving up on you but rather is trying to protect you from harm that might affect you badly. Your doctor then will concentrate on alleviating any symptoms that you have.

96. What is best supportive care?

Supportive care is care concentrated on treating and controlling symptoms. It is an active approach and you will still see your doctor regularly. You will be discussing pain control, nutrition, abdominal distention or leg swelling, if any, jaundice, and other symptoms or concerns that you might have. Controlling those symptoms will allow you to maintain some functional level at this stage of your disease. You should use this time to visit your family and friends, visit places you like, enjoy your hobbies, and attend religious services. Keeping a positive and hopeful attitude is the key to succeed through this period of time.

97. What is hospice?

If your medical condition worsens, you may become debilitated and need a great deal of help and support. This can be provided through **hospice** care. Hospice is a global care approach that addresses medical, physical, emotional, social, and spiritual needs for patients with advanced-stage disease. This care can be provided at home, especially if your family is around and is able and ready to provide the physical care. You will be visited by a hospice registered nurse and possibly a hospice care physician on a regular basis and as frequently as is necessary. The regular assessments will ensure that you remain comfortable and that all of your needs are addressed. The hospice care team will consult regularly with your doctor. If necessary, you may be provided with a home health aide to assist you with your physical needs, such as bathing. Although the hospice caring team will be present at your home for only a few hours a day, it will be available 24 hours a day, 7 days a week if an emergency arises.

Hospice

A facility or program that provides medical, emotional, and spiritual support for terminally ill patients at an inpatient facility or at the patient's home.

You also may have hospice care provided at a hospice facility as an inpatient because of personal wishes, family members who need to go to work, or if you require strenuous care that your family members cannot provide. At this time of illness, you still can have quality time with your family and loved ones at an inpatient hospice facility with extended visiting hours. Meanwhile, the staff will provide all of the care that you need.

You are entitled to hospice care after you and your doctor decide not to pursue any further active care, such as chemotherapy. If your illness appears life threatening at this time, your doctor may recommend hospice. A hospice program may include palliative care. Additional information is available at www.hospiceinfo.org. Some hospice facilities provide palliative care or specific spiritual care. You can discuss with your doctor what options are available or visit the website of the National Hospice and Palliative Care Organization at www.nhpco.org.

If your medical condition worsens, you may become debilitated and need a great deal of help and support.

In addition to giving top-notch care for my father, the hospice provided much needed relief for us, the family. They took care of all of the little things, such as checking up on him during the night, changing his position in bed, and making sure that he took his pain medication. They allowed my mother to rest and recuperate.

At the time, I hated the idea of the hospice because it forced me to come to grips that the care was palliative only and that my father's condition was terminal. However, I could not hate the hospice itself. The nurses were always friendly and attentive, and the condition of the facility was much nicer than the hospital. The hospice that we found was about 10 miles from my sister's home. After 3 days there, my father expressed his wishes to be in a more familiar environment; thus, the hospice helped us transport him to my sister's house, where we could be with him during his final days.

98. What are advanced directives?

Considering the advanced nature of your cancer, you may want to direct your caring team in advance about your wishes. **Advanced directives** are legal documents that are made to protect your wishes and to make sure that those are granted. The two basic forms of advanced directives are a living will and a **healthcare proxy**.

Advanced directives

Patient's wishes that he or she expresses in advance in regard to terminal illness.

Healthcare proxy

Person assigned by or designated for a patient to help make medical decisions in the case the patient's condition does not allow him or her to do so.

Cardiopulmonary resuscitation

An emergency procedure in which cardiac massage, artificial respiration, and drugs are used to regain and maintain heart and lung function.

In a living will, you may state specific instructions that relate to your medical care in case you are unable to communicate them. It should state clearly your wishes in case your heart stops beating or you stop breathing. Your doctor may offer a short version of a living will that addresses those two issues. In case of advanced cancer, your medical condition may worsen enough that your heart and lung stop working and die. You may ask for **cardiopulmonary resuscitation** and have compressions on your chest, electric shock applied to your heart, medications infused to speed your heart, a plastic tube inserted down your throat, and connection made to a breathing machine. In the case of advanced cancer, these heroic interventions are more likely to fail. If anything, they may be tormenting, painful, and undignifying to you and your family. In those instances, your doctor may recommend that you have a do-not-resuscitate (DNR)/ do-not-intubate (DNI) order. Of course, you have the full right to refuse and still ask for those interventions. Have an open and frank discussion with your doctor about DNR/DNI orders to make sure that you understand them fully. Discuss those wishes in advance and do not leave them until late in your disease. When you are comfortable and do not feel pushed, you are more likely to make a rational decision. Remember that a DNR/DNI order does not limit your access to medical care in any way. You still may be receiving chemotherapy but already have stated your wishes about end-of-life issues.

Your living will also might include wishes that relate to drawing blood, giving blood, feeding, **dialysis**, and the like. Make sure that all of this is discussed fully with your doctor. Generally, your doctor will not recommend any invasive measures, except if they truly will improve your survival. Otherwise, he or she will guide you to make a decision that would improve your comfort. Remember that some times in medicine, doing less is doing more.

Dialysis
Clearing blood of toxins by passing it through machines, in case of kidney failure.

The other part of the advanced directive is to assign a healthcare proxy. You may need to do that, and it is highly recommended either because some states do not recognize living wills, or because some decisions not previously discussed with you need to be made while you are asleep, unconscious, or simply unable to make them. In those instances, your healthcare proxy (also called a health surrogate, a medical proxy, or a medical power of attorney) will act on your behalf and make those decisions.

A healthcare proxy should be someone whom you trust and someone you know and believe will make decisions based on your wishes stated and unstated. This can be a family member or a friend. Make sure to inform your healthcare proxy of interest about your wish to assign them. Make sure that he or she is comfortable with that decision, and if so, make sure to lead a candid and honest discussion about your wishes. It is important that you inform your friends and family about who is your healthcare proxy in order to avoid any unnecessary conflict that may arise at some tense moments. You can discuss healthcare proxy issues with your caring team, the social worker, patient representative, or your lawyer.

A healthcare proxy should be someone whom you trust and someone you know and believe will make decisions based on your wishes stated and unstated.

99. What should I do to prepare to die? Where is hope?

Although death is a fearful reality, preparing for it might help erase that fear and make it more of a transitional phase that is an integral part of our life cycle. You should never believe that thinking of death means giving up, especially your sense of purpose. It is rather an opportunity that helps you shape how your life will end. The earlier that you prepare, the better, because you do not want to feel pressured or disappointed if things do not go the way you wish.

Clear your financial issues. Work with your attorney, accountant, and your family. You may need to write a will, especially if you have family who is financially dependent on you. Sort out your financial plan and keep your attorney's name and contacts available. Also, keep all legal, financial, or health documents organized for easier access.

Visit with your loved ones, family, friends, and colleagues. Talk to people who live far away. If you are troubled by any unresolved issues with somebody, work on sorting them out. Indicate to whom you want to give any valuable items you have. Collectibles and photographs are memories that will celebrate your life and may be passed from one generation to another. You may wish to prepare some aspects of your funeral. This is a celebration of your life and an important closure for everybody.

The biggest fear that remains is leaving your loved ones behind, especially children. See them as often as you can. Prepare an album of photos about moments of your life that you would like to share with them. Leave any scrapbooks or diaries for them.

As you can imagine, you still might be busy even close to your death. Remember and recite to yourself your dearest moments. You will notice that you are abundant with life.

One of my closest friends, Francis, lost his father to liver cancer shortly before I did. He told me the best advice ever. Tell your father you love him for everything he has done. Do it early and often. I am glad I listened to him. In the few days before he passed away, my father had trouble speaking due to encephalopathy, and thus, I could only be there to comfort him. It is very important to communicate as much as possible before the illness becomes too advanced.

100. Where can I find additional information?

Throughout the book, several other resources were mentioned that might help you to get additional information or answers to your questions. In this computer age, the Internet is a great resource to many aspects of your liver cancer. Generally, the information is periodically updated.

You have to exert caution, however, because some Internet sites may have information that is not verified. Always check with your healthcare team if you are in doubt. Chat rooms could be another resource that helps you to share your experience and exchange information. Remember, however, that no two patients are alike; thus, treat this information critically before acting on it. A comprehensive cancer center can have many resources available to you as well. Always make sure to ask because you will be amazed at how much care and support are available.

Glossary

A

Abdominal distention: Bulging of the belly.

Ablation: The destruction of a tumor without actually removing it. Examples include heating (radiofrequency ablation), freezing (cryotherapy), injecting a toxic substance such as ethanol or chemotherapy, or decreasing its blood supply, as in hepatic artery embolization.

Abscess: A collection of pus.

Acupuncture: A Chinese medical procedure in which fine needles are placed through the skin to relieve pain or for other treatment reasons.

Acute viral hepatitis: An active infection caused by a hepatitis virus.

Adjuvant therapy: A form of therapy that will help prevent the recurrence of cancer after a potentially curative treatment such as surgery.

Advanced directives: Patient's wishes that he or she expresses in advance in regard to terminal illness.

Aflatoxins: A group of molds that contaminate stored food supplies and may lead to cirrhosis and ultimately liver cancer.

Alcohol injection: Inserting alcohol through a needle into a tumor. This technique is widely used to treat small hepatomas. Alcohol is directly toxic to the tumor.

Alpha-fetoprotein: A blood marker that may be elevated in primary liver cancer.

Alcoholic liver disease: Liver cirrhosis caused by excessive alcohol ingestion.

Alternative medicine: Medical practices (e.g., herbal medicine) that do not follow Western medicine guidelines and may lack scientific proof for their effectiveness.

Ammonia: A body of excreted substances that normally is broken down by the liver.

Anesthesia: Medication that puts someone to sleep and/or reduces pain.

Anesthesiologist: A doctor who specializes in the delivery of anesthesia.

Antibiotics: Medications used to fight infections.

Aorta: The largest artery in the body. It originates from the heart, and its branches supply the entire body with blood containing oxygen.

Arteriography: A radiologic test that demonstrates the artery branches of a person. The technique is performed by an interventional radiologist. Typically, a small tube is inserted into the patient's leg during the procedure. A contrast agent is injected, and x-rays are then taken to reveal the arteries. Arteriography is used to identify the artery branches that supply a tumor during hepatic artery embolization.

Ascites: An abnormal accumulation of fluid in the abdomen.

B

Bile: A collection of salts and proteins that is made by the liver and carried by the bile duct to the gallbladder and the intestine. Bile is green and gives feces their brown color.

Bilirubin: A component of bile that comes from the breakdown of red blood cells.

Biologic therapy: Novel agents aimed at specific targets used to treat cancer.

Biopsy: The physical sampling of a piece of tissue. In patients with a suspected tumor, a biopsy is used to determine whether the patient has a cancer and what type of tumor it is. A biopsy is generally performed by passing a needle through the skin into a tumor.

Bone marrow: Substance that fills the bone inner cavities and is the source of red blood cells, white blood cells, and platelets.

Brachytherapy: Radiation therapy that is applied within the body cavity.

C

Cancer: The uncontrolled replication of cells that leads to abnormal growth that may invade local organs or tissues or may travel to other places in the body.

Cardiopulmonary resuscitation: An emergency procedure in which cardiac massage, artificial respiration, and drugs are used to regain and maintain heart and lung function.

Cells: The smallest structural unit of a living organism that is capable of functioning independently.

Chemotherapy: Chemical agents that are used to treat cancer.

Child-Pugh score: A score used to assess the level of cirrhosis.

Cholangiocarcinoma: Cancer of the bile ducts.

Chronic viral hepatitis: Continuous state of infection during which the liver continues to be inflamed and may ultimately cause cirrhosis and cancer.

Cirrhosis: Condition in which normal liver tissue is replaced with scarred tissue. It is often associated with varied levels of loss of liver functions.

Clinical trial: A research study that answers many of the questions regarding newly discovered therapies.

Coma: Loss of consciousness that may occur when the liver is no longer working well.

Complementary medicine (same as alternative medicine): Medical practices (e.g., herbal medicine) that do not follow Western medicine guidelines and that may lack a scientific proof for their effectiveness.

Computed tomography (CT) scan: A form of x-ray images in which acquired images are constructed by computer to form cross-sectional images of the body.

Creatinine: A substance usually excreted from the body through urine. It is used to help assess kidney function.

Cryotherapy: A form of therapy that uses cold temperature to kill cancer cells.

Cytotoxic drugs: Chemical substances that are used as chemotherapy to kill cancer cells.

Depression: A sad state of mind characterized by feeling tired, with an inability to concentrate, an inability to sleep, a decreased appetite, guilt, and thoughts of death. Although it may be a psychiatric illness, it also may occur in patients facing a serious illness, such as primary liver cancer or other forms of cancer.

D

Diabetes: A disease condition in which the body is unable to control sugar levels. In some instances, diabetes may lead to multiple complications and other diseases, and possibly primary liver cancer.

Dialysis: Clearing blood of toxins by passing it through machines, in case of kidney failure.

Diuretics (water pills): Drugs that increase the discharge of urine.

E

Echocardiogram: A test for the heart in which pictures and functional values of the heart are obtained using ultrasound.

Edema: An abnormal accumulation of fluid in the extremities.

Electrocardiogram: An electrical tracing of the heart.

Encephalopathy: An altered sense of consciousness. It may occur when the liver is not working well. The patient may seemed confused or have inappropriate social behavior. It may vary in severity from day to day.

Endoscopy: A procedure performed by a gastroenterologist. A tube is placed into your mouth while you are lightly sedated. The doctor can then look at the inside of the stomach and the first part of the intestine to search for dilated blood vessels (varices), ulcers, or gastritis.

External beam radiation: Radiation therapy that is aimed at a specific site in the body and delivered from outside of the body through the skin.

F

Fatigue: Physical tiredness.

Fatty liver: Condition in which fat accumulates in the liver because of a liver illness caused by one of several diseases (e.g., viral hepatitis).

Fibrolamellar hepatocellular carcinoma: A variant of hepatoma that occurs typically in young adults. It generally has a more favorable outcome and is not associated with underlying liver disease.

Foley catheter: A tube that is placed into the bladder to monitor precisely the urine output of a patient.

Four-phase CT: A CT scan that evaluates the liver in four phases as the blood flows through it.

Fungus: A type of organism that can cause an infection.

G

Gallbladder: A storage tank for bile. It is attached to the liver. It squeezes the bile into your intestine when you eat a fatty meal.

Gastritis: Inflammation of the inside lining of the stomach.

Gastroenterologist: A doctor who specializes in the treatment of diseases that affect the gastrointestinal system, including the liver, stomach, and pancreas.

Gene: A genetic sequence made of DNA that encodes for a specific protein.

Genotype: The genetic constitution of a specific virus or any organism.

H

Healthcare proxy: Person assigned by, or designated for, a patient to help make medical decisions in the case the patient's condition does not allow him or her to do so.

Hematoma: A collection of blood.

Hemochromatosis: A hereditary disease that leads to excessive accumulation of iron in the body and may cause liver disease and ultimately primary liver cancer.

Hepatic artery: The blood vessel that carries oxygenated blood to the liver.

Hepatic artery embolization (chemoembolization): The injection of microscopic particles (either attached to a chemotherapy drug or not) into the branches of the hepatic artery in order to ablate or destroy a liver tumor. The treatment works by blocking the blood supply to the tumor and, when chemotherapy is used, by delivering chemotherapy to the tumor.

Hepatitis: Inflammation of the liver. It may be caused by a variety of agents, including viruses, excessive alcohol use, metabolic diseases, and environmental toxins.

Hepatobiliary surgeon: A doctor who specializes in the surgical and ablative treatments of liver, gallbladder, bile duct, and pancreas tumors.

Hepatoblastoma: A rare type of primary liver cancer that occurs in children.

Hepatocellular cancer: A type of primary liver cancer that originates in hepatocytes; a type of liver cell.

Hepatocellular carcinoma: Cancer of the liver cells, a type of primary liver cancer.

Hepatocytes: Liver cells.

Hepatologist: A liver disease specialist.

Hepatoma: Short name for hepatocellular cancer.

Homeopathy: Treating disease with small amounts of treatments that in large amounts in healthy people may produce symptoms of the same disease. This is a medical practice that is based on resemblance between the drug and the disease.

Hospice: A facility or program that provides medical, emotional, and spiritual support for terminally ill patients at an inpatient facility or at the patient's home.

Human immunodeficiency virus (HIV): A virus that destroys helper cells of the immune system that usually fight infections and may lead to AIDS.

I

Immune system: An intricate body system that protects people against foreign organisms or toxins that may cause disease.

Inferior vena cava: A large vein that is supplied by multiple veins from the lower parts of the body and helps bring the blood back to the heart.

Institutional review board: A collective board that oversees all clinical trials. The board generally includes doctors, researchers, lawyers, administrators, pharmacists, and patients' advocates.

Integrative medicine: A discipline that is used to treat patients using modern science and alternative medicine.

Interventional radiologist: A doctor who specializes in performing procedures under radiologic (ultrasound, x-ray, or CT scan) guidance such as tumor biopsies, hepatic artery embolization, or a mediport.

Intestine: The part of the gastrointestinal tract between the stomach and rectum. The intestine helps digest food and regulate water, certain vitamins, and salts of the body.

J

Jaundice: Yellowish discoloration of the skin and eyes caused by accumulation of bilirubin.

K

Kidneys: Two organs located in the abdomen that are responsible for water and electrolytes balance, and that help excrete body metabolites through urine.

L

Lamivudine Entecavir, Adefovir-dipivoxil: Antivirus drugs commonly used against hepatitis B.

Laparoscopy: A procedure that is done under general anesthesia and performed by a surgeon in which the inside of the abdomen can be examined through a few small incisions.

Liver: An organ located in the upper right-hand side of the abdomen; responsible for making proteins and removing toxins and wastes from the body.

Liver capsule: The outside lining of the liver. It is the only part of the liver that can trigger a sensation of pain.

Liver resection: The surgical removal of all or a portion of the liver.

Local anesthetic: Numbing medication that is injected directly at the site where a procedure is to be performed.

Lymph nodes: Small bodies along the lymphatic system that supply a special kind of fighter white blood cells called lymphocytes to the bloodstream. They are also responsible for removing bacteria and foreign particles from the lymph. Lymph nodes may be invaded by cancer and may also help transmit cancer to other sites of the body. Lymph nodes are also known as lymph glands.

M

Magnetic resonance imaging (MRI): A form of radiologic imaging that uses magnetic fields to produce electronic images of the inner parts of the human body.

Mediport: A half-dollar sized, round well that is connected to a tube that is used for the delivery of medication within a vein. The entire apparatus sits underneath the skin and is inserted during a small procedure.

MELD (Model for End-Stage Liver Disease): A mathematical equation that is used to prioritize patients for liver transplantation based on their laboratory values.

Metabolic diseases: Diseases in which the metabolism of a certain product may be impaired. They are usually genetically inherited.

Metastasis: The spread of cancer beyond its primary location.

N

Naturopathy: The science that uses herbs and herb products as a form of therapy against disease.

Nausea: The feeling of sickness in the stomach with an urge to vomit.

Neoadjuvant therapy: Therapy that is given before surgical removal of a cancer, aiming at reducing its size and rendering it more resectable.

Nerve: A type of tissue in the body that can transmit sensations such as pain, pressure, or temperature.

Nonalcoholic fatty liver disease: Disease that leads to the development of fatty liver by injuries other than excessive alcohol use.

Nonalcoholic steatohepatitis: Progression from nonalcoholic fatty liver disease to cirrhosis and potentially cancer.

Nonsteroidal anti-inflammatory drugs: A form of medication that controls pain and inflammation that is not part of the steroid family.

O

Oncologists: Medical doctor specialists who treat cancer.

P

Partial hepatectomy: The surgical removal of part of the liver.

Pathologist: A doctor who specializes in the diagnosis of diseases of the body by evaluating biopsies from the disease site, like cancer.

Pathology laboratory: The section of the hospital in which a pathologist works and where tissue specimens are analyzed.

Pathology report: A typed report issued by a pathologist that describes the results of the analysis of a biopsy or surgical specimen.

Pathology slides: 3×1–inch glass slides on which tissue from a biopsy or a surgical specimen is placed.

Peripheral edema: Excessive accumulation of fluids in the legs that leads to swelling.

Platelets: Pieces of cells that float in the blood and promote clotting where necessary.

Pneumonia: A lung infection.

Portal hypertension: Increased pressure within the veins of the liver, which can lead to poor liver function, increased size of the spleen, and consequently, a low platelet count, or varices (dilated veins of the stomach or esophagus).

Portal vein: A blood vessel that carries blood from the intestines to within the liver.

Primary liver cancer: Cancer that originates within the liver.

Prognostic: A blood test, sign, or other element that helps predict the likely course of the cancer.

Proteins: Essential body substances that include enzymes, hormones, antibodies, and other substances that are critical for the functioning of the human body.

Prothrombin: A protein produced by the liver that helps blood to clot.

Protocol: A detailed description of all of the rules and conditions that govern a clinical trial. A protocol is the ultimate reference for a clinical trial.

Pump: A pump system used to deliver chemotherapy at a fixed rate and for a specific period of time.

R

Radiation: A ray of powerful energy that is emitted from a radioactive material.

Radiation hepatitis: Inflammatory damage to the liver that may be caused by radiation therapy.

Radiation therapy: Treatment against cancer that uses radiation as a form of energy to kill cancer cells.

Radiofrequency ablation: A form of tumor ablation that relies on heating to destroy tumor cells. It may be performed by inserting a metal probe through the skin into a liver tumor. Alternatively, it may be performed at the time of laparoscopy or laparotomy (open surgical exploration).

Radiologists: Doctors who specialize in interpreting x-rays, CT scans, MRIs, and other radiologic tests.

Red blood cells: Cells that carry oxygen and carbon dioxide. They are red because of their high load of iron, which is essential to their function.

Rejection: The process by which the body refuses a donated transplanted liver and regards it as foreign.

S

Screening: Studies and evaluations that attempt to identify a predisease state or an early form of disease, aiming at controlling it before it becomes advanced.

Secondary liver cancer: Cancers that started in other organs of the body and have traveled to the liver.

Spleen: An organ located in the upper left part of the abdomen that filters toxic foreign substances from the blood. In case of liver failure, the spleen may enlarge.

Staging system: A set of definitions that allows physicians to define the extent of a certain cancer and recommend therapy accordingly.

T

Thrombosis: The formation of clots.

Tolerance: The body's need for an increased dose of a certain medication to obtain the same effect.

Transplantation: The removal of a patient's entire liver and replacement with part or all of the liver from another person. The other person may be alive (live donor) or just deceased (cadaveric donor).

Triphasic CT: A CT scan that evaluates the liver at three phases as the blood flows through it.

Tumor: A cancerous growth.

U

Ulcer: A lesion of the stomach that results from inflammation and may bleed.

Ultrasound: The use of ultrasonic waves to view images of an internal body structure.

V

Variceal bleed: An actively bleeding varix, which is a dilated vein.

Varix: An abnormally swollen vein that is prone to bleed.

Viral hepatitis: Inflammatory condition of the liver caused by an infection with a hepatitis virus.

W

White blood cells: Cells that help fight infection.

Wilson's disease: An inherited disease of impaired copper metabolism.

Y

Yttrium-90 microspheres: Small beads tagged with radioactive yttrium that are delivered into the liver and lodge inside the small arteries to deliver their anticancer therapeutic effect.

Index

Note: Page numbers followed by *b*, *f*, or *t* indicate material in boxes, figures, or tables, respectively.

A

abdominal distention, 22
ablation, 40. *See also* radiofrequency ablation
  tumor, 63
abscess, 65
acetaminophen (Tylenol), 102, 103
acupuncture, 90
acute viral hepatitis, 7
adjuvant therapy
  after liver resection, 53–54
  before liver resection, 54–55
Adriamycin (doxorubicin), 54, 84–85
advanced directives, 118–119
Advil, 102
aflatoxins, 15
AFP. *See* alpha-fetoprotein
ALBI scoring system, 29
alcohol injection, 40, 40*b*, 67–68
alcohol use, liver and, 12
alcoholic liver disease, 12
Aldactone (spironolactone), 106
alpha-fetoprotein (AFP), 19–20, 25–26, 69, 74
alpha-1 antitrypsin deficiency, 14*b*
alternative medicine, 89–91
American with Disabilities Act, 115
ammonia, 111
anesthesia, 44
anesthesiologist, 47
antibiotics, 65, 81
aorta, 64
arteriography, 59
ascites, 22, 23*b*, 51, 106
  management of, 107
Aspergillus flavus, 15
Aspergillus parasiticus, 15
Atarax, 110
ataxia telangiectasia, 14*b*

B

Barraclude, 9
BCLC system, 29
Benadryl, 24, 99, 110
bile, 2, 50
  mechanical blockage of, 100–101
biliary atresia, 14*b*
biliary leak, 61
bilirubin, 58, 110
biologic therapy, 26, 38, 40*b*, 68–69
  assessing response of, 74–76
  side effects of, 69–73
biopsy, 9
  for diagnosis, 26–27
  needle, 27
bland embolization, 64
bleeding
  after liver transplantation, 61
  ways to stop, 109
blocked bile duct, fixing of, 100–101
blood pressure, 72
brachytherapy, 87
Budd-Chiari syndrome, 14*b*

C

Cabometyx (cabozantinib), 69, 72
cadaveric liver, 57–58
  transplantation, 60
cancer, 3
cardiopulmonary resuscitation, 118
cells, 3
Centerwatch, 79
chemoembolization, 66. *See also* hepatic artery embolization
chemotherapy, 26, 40*b*, 80–82
  drugs, 84–86
  liver pump, 86
  side effects of, 82–84
Child-Pugh scoring system, 29, 33
chimeric antigen receptors (CAR) T cells, 80
cholangiocarcinoma, 4
chronic hepatitis B, 8–10
chronic hepatitis C, 10–12
chronic viral hepatitis, 6
cirrhosis
  complications of, 23*b*
  liver cancer, 22–23
    treatment and, 32–33
  quality and length of life and, 32–33
cisplatin, 54, 85
citrullinemia, 14*b*
clinical trial, 54, 77–79
  learning and selection of, 79–80
CLIP scoring system, 29
Coalition of National Cancer Cooperative Groups, 79
Colace, 104
coma, 110
complementary medicine, 89–91
computed tomography (CT), 19, 24
  assessing response of biologic/targeted therapies and immunotherapy, 74–76
congenital hepatic fibrosis, 14*b*
creatinine, 58
cryotherapy, 40*b*, 41, 66–67
CT. *See* computed tomography
CUPI scoring system, 29
Cyramza (ramicirumab), 69, 73
cytotoxic drugs, 80–81

D

daclatasvir (Daklinza), 11
death, preparation for, 120–121
depression, 36
diabetes, 6
  obesity, liver cancer and, 13
dialysis, 119
diarrhea, 71
diet, 97–98
diuretics, 51, 106
do-not-resuscitate (DNR)/do-not-intubate (DNI) order, 118
Duphala (lactulose), 111

E

echocardiogram, 47
edema, 106
  management of, 107
elbasvir, 11
electrocardiogram, 47
embolization. *See also specific embolization*
  side effects of, 65
  systemic therapy with, 66
emotions management after diagnosis, 35–36
encephalopathy, 23, 110
endoscopy, 59
esophageal varices, 108–109
external beam radiation, 87

F

familial cholestatic cirrhosis, 14*b*
familial polyposis coli, 14*b*
fatigue, 7, 71–72, 101–102. *See also* mental fatigue
fatty liver, 12

Fentanyl, 103
fetal alcohol syndrome, 14*b*
fibrolamellar carcinoma. *See* fibrolamellar hepatocellular carcinoma
fibrolamellar hepatocellular carcinoma, 4
5-fluorouracil, 54, 84–85
Foley catheter, 48
FOLFOX, 84–85, 86
four-phase CT scan, 75
fungus, 15
furosemide (Lasix), 106

G

galactosemia, 14*b*
gallbladder, 4, 49–50
gastritis, 51
gastroenterologist, 100
genes, 28
genetic testing, 28
genotype, 11
glecaprevir, 11
glycogen storage disease, types 1 and 3, 14*b*
grazoprevir (Zepatier), 11

H

hand-foot skin reaction, 70–71
Harvoni (sofosbuvir), 11
HCC. *See* hepatocellular cancer
healthcare proxy, 118, 119
hematoma, 65
hemochromatosis, 13–14, 14*b*
hepatic artery, 45
  clotting, 61
  embolization, 40*b*, 41, 63, 64–66
hepatitis, 6. *See also specific hepatitis*
  acute viral, 7
  chronic viral, 6
  radiation, 87
  recurrent, 62
  from recurring and infecting new liver, 63
  viral, 7–8
hepatitis A, 7–8
hepatitis B, 7–10
hepatitis C, 7–8, 10–12
hepatobiliary surgeons, 42
hepatoblastoma, 4
hepatocellular cancer (HCC), 3
  cirrhosis and, 7, 7*f*
  treatments for, 40*b*
  in world, 6
hepatocytes, 3, 4
hepatologist, 33
hepatoma, 4. *See also* hepatocellular cancer
Hepsera, 9
hereditary tyrosinemia, 14*b*
HIV. *See* human immunodeficiency virus
homeopathy, 90
hospice, 116–117
human immunodeficiency virus (HIV), 58–59
hypertension, portal, 23, 23*b*, 106

I

immune system, 62
immunotherapy
  assessing response of, 74–76
  defined, 73–74
  side effects of, 73–74
improved survival, 69
infection
  after liver transplantation, 62
  new liver, 63
inferior vena cava, 45
informed consent, 78
institutional review board, 77
insurance coverage, 36–38
integrative medicine, 33
interferon, 11, 54, 85
Internet, 92–93, 121
interventional radiologist, 51, 64

intestine, 2
investigational biologic therapy, 40*b*
investigational chemotherapy, 40*b*
investigational targeted therapy, 40*b*

J

jaundice, 7, 22–23, 23*b*, 99–100, 109–110

K

kidneys, 23

L

lactulose (Duphala), 104, 111
Lamivudine, 9
laparoscopy, 48, 67
Lasix (furosemide), 106
ledipasvir, 11
lenvatinib (Lenvima), 68–69, 72–73, 75, 76
leucovorin, 84
liver
  alcohol use affecting, 12
  described, 2
  destruction, 109–110
  if does not function as well, 76
  functions of, 2*b*
  inherited metabolic diseases and, 13–14
  new, source of, 57–58
  segments of, 46*f*
liver cancer
  cirrhosis and, 22–23, 32–33
  described, 4
  diagnosis of, 24–26
    biopsy for, 26–27
    insurance and financial concerns, 36–38
    management of emotions after, 35–36
    second opinion, 33–35
  diet for, 97–98
  doctors suggestion to stop therapies, 115
  environmental factors causing, 15
  factors for determining tumor can be removed, 44–45, 46*f*
  genetic diseases causing, 14*b*
  obesity, diabetes, and, 13
  options if tumor returns, 55
  person at risk for developing, 6
  recommendations if no treatment performed, 91–92
  staging, 28–29
  survival of person with, 32
  symptoms of, 22
  transmission of, 114
  treatment. *See also specific therapies*
    decision making regarding, 96–97
    liver resection. *See* liver resection
    liver transplantation. *See* liver transplantation
    options for, 40–41, 40*b*
  types of, 2*t*, 3–4
  ways to reduce risks, 15–16
  work while getting treated, 114–115
liver capsule, 19
liver pump chemotherapy, 86
liver resection, 40, 40*b*
  adjuvant therapy for, 53–55
  complications of, 50–51
  incisions for, 49*f*
  outcome of, 52–53
  pathology report, 52
  preparations for, 46–48
  things happening after, 50
  things happening during, 48–50
liver transplantation, 40, 40*b*
  cadaveric, 60
  complications of, 61–62
  evaluation for, 58–59
  living related donor, 60–61
  outcomes of, 62–63

preventing cancer from returning after, 62–63
reason and time for performing, 55–57
things happening while waiting, 59
living related donor liver, 58
transplantation, 60–61
local anesthetic, 27
lymph nodes, 25

M

magnesium citrate, 104
magnetic resonance imaging (MRI), 19, 20, 24
assessing response of biologic/targeted therapies and immunotherapy, 74–76
Mavyret (pibrentasvir), 11–12
Medicaid, 37, 38
mediport, 86, 98–99
MELD scoring system, 29
mental confusion, 23*b*
mental fatigue, 101–102
metabolic diseases, 6
inherited, 13–14
metastasis, 3, 88
Miralax, 104
model for end-stage liver disease (MELD), 58
Motrin, 102
MRI. *See* magnetic resonance imaging
MS Contin, 103
multi-disciplinary care, 34, 41–43

N

NAFLD. *See* nonalcoholic fatty liver disease
NASH. *See* nonalcoholic steatohepatitis
National Cancer Institute, 79
National Comprehensive Cancer Center Network, 84
National Hospice and Palliative Care Organization, 117
National Institutes of Health, 89
naturopathy, 90
needle biopsy, 27
neo-adjuvant therapy, 54, 85
nerve, 19
neurofibromatosis, 14*b*
new liver
hepatitis from recurring and infecting, 63
source of, 57–58
Nexavar (sorafenib), 54, 66, 68–69, 71–73, 76, 96, 108
next generation sequencing (NGS) test, 28
nivolumab (Opdivo), 73, 74, 76
nonalcoholic fatty liver disease (NAFLD), 6, 13
nonalcoholic steatohepatitis (NASH), 13
nonsteroidal anti-inflammatory drugs (NSAIDs), 102

O

obesity, liver cancer, diabetes and, 13
Okuda scoring system, 29
ombitasvir, 12
oncologists, 29
Opdivo (nivolumab), 73, 74, 76
open laparotomy, 67
opiates, 103
side effects of, 103–104
oxaliplatin, 84
oxycodone, 103
oxycontin, 103

P

pain, 102–104
palliative care, 117

paritaprevir, 12
partial hepatectomy. *See* liver resection
pathologist, 27
pathology
  laboratory, 27
  report, 28
    information in, 52
  slides, 27
Percocet, 103
peripheral edema, 22, 23*b*, 106
PIAF, 55, 85
pibrentasvir (Mavyret), 11–12
platelets, 83
  low count, 107–108
pneumonia, 51
porphyria cutanea tarda, 14*b*
portal hypertension, 23, 23*b*, 106
portal vein, 45
  embolization, 45
preadmission testing, 47
primary biliary cirrhosis, 14*b*
primary liver cancer, 2*t*, 3–4
  new drugs and treatment approaches for, 80
primary liver nonfunction, 61
prognostic value, 26
proteins, 2
prothrombin, 58
protocols, 77
pump, 86

R

radiation hepatitis, 87
radiation therapy, 19, 86–88
  side effects of, 89
  Yttrium-90 microspheres, 88–89
radioembolization, 63
radiofrequency ablation (RFA), 40, 40*b*, 63, 66–67
radiologist, 26
  interventional, 64
ramicirumab (Cyramza), 68–69, 73
red blood cells, 83
regorafenib (Stivarga), 68–69, 71–72
rejection, 62
RFA. *See* radiofrequency ablation
ribavarin, 11
ritonavir (Technivie), 12

S

screening, 10
  entailing of, 19–20
  frequency of, 20
  of person with risk factors, 18
  reason for, 18–19
  things should be done after suggestion, 20
second opinion, 33–35
secondary liver cancer, 2*t*, 4
Senekot, 104
situs inversus, 14*b*
Social Security, 37
Social Security disability, 37
sofosbuvir (Harvoni, Sovaldi), 11
sorafenib (Nexavar), 54, 66, 68–69, 71–73, 76, 96, 108
Sovaldi (sofosbuvir), 11
spironolactone (Aldactone), 106
spleen, 107
staging system, 28–29
steroids, 24
Stivarga (regorafenib), 68–69, 71–73
stomach varices, 108–109
supportive care, 33, 40*b*, 115–116

T

targeted therapy, 40*b*, 68–69
  assessing response of, 74–76
  side effects of, 69–73
Technivie (ritonavir), 12
theraspheres. *See* Yttrium-90 microspheres
thrombosis, 61
tolerance, 103
transplantation, 7
triphasic CT, 75

tumor, 3
  ablation, 63
Tylenol (acetaminophen), 102, 103
tyrosine kinase inhibitors, 68

U

ulcer, 51
ultrasound, 19, 20
  assessing response of biologic/targeted therapies and immunotherapy, 74–76
United Network for Organ Sharing (UNOS), 57
U.S. Department of Justice, 115
U.S. Department of Labor Medical Leave Act of 1993, 114

V

variceal bleeding, 23, 23*b*
varices, 51
  esophageal, 108–109
  stomach, 108–109
Veterans Affairs Department, 37
viral hepatitis, 7–8

W

water pills. *See* diuretics
white blood cells, 83
Wilson's disease, 14*b*

X

X-ray machine, 64

Y

Yttrium-90 microspheres, 88–89

Z

Zepatier (grazoprevir), 11